D0701385

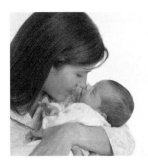

Praise for
Spanish for Breastfeeding Support

"Communication is key to helping Spanish-speaking mothers succeed with breastfeeding. This resource will make that communication so much easier."

- Jack Newman, MD, author of *The Ultimate Book of Breastfeeding Answers*

"This book provides outstanding teaching methods for learning Spanish, with real world breastfeeding scenarios and helpful exercises for practice. It will be a great tool for medical Spanish teachers, lactation consultants, nurses, doctors and others serving Spanish-speaking mothers."

- Mariana Achugar, Associate Professor of Spanish and Second Language Acquisition, Carnegie Mellon University

"Communicating breastfeeding information in Spanish is becoming more and more necessary and important. I'm very excited about this wonderful new resource for people who work in breastfeeding support!"

- Diana West, IBCLC, author of *The Breastfeeding Mother's Guide to Making More Milk*

"As a Latina working with Spanish-speaking mothers, I value the accurate translation in this book, as well as the use of common expressions and phrases. This book is an excellent tool for effective lactation support."

- Jackie Aguas, IBCLC, Lactation Coordinator, Merced, California WIC

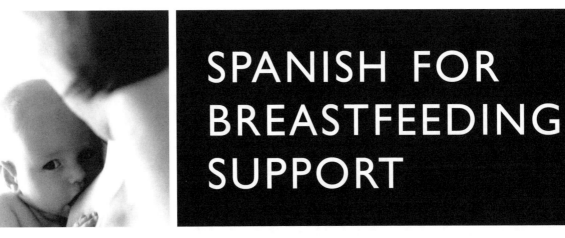

SPANISH FOR BREASTFEEDING SUPPORT

A SELF-GUIDED COURSE TO HELP YOU SUPPORT BREASTFEEDING MOTHERS IN SPANISH

Diana B. Glick, M.A. and Tanya M. Lieberman, IBCLC | www.spanishforbreastfeedingsupport.com

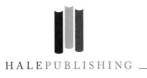

HALEPUBLISHING

1712 N. Forest St. • Amarillo, Texas 79106 | © Copyright 2009 All rights reserved.

©Copyright 2009
Hale Publishing, L.P.
1712 N. Forest St.
Amarillo, TX 79106 USA
www.iBreastfeeding.com

(806)376-9900 (phone)
(800)378-1317 (toll-free)
(806)376-9901 (fax)
(+1-806)376-9900 (international)

Printed in Canada

Illustrator: Noah Barrett

ISBN: 978-0-9815257-8-5

Library of Congress Number: 2009921417

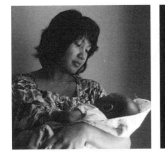

TABLE OF CONTENTS

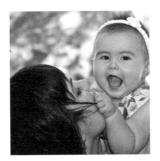

THE AUTHORS ARE GRATEFUL
TO THE FOLLOWING INDIVIDUALS FOR
REVIEWING DRAFTS OF THIS BOOK
AND OFFERING THEIR EXCELLENT ADVICE

Lori Feldman-Winter, MD, MPH

Diana Molina, LLL leader

Zilkia Escuerdo, WIC Breastfeeding Peer Counselor

Angela White, J.D., LLL leader

Joanna Patraw, RD, IBCLC

Mary Carey, RN, IBCLC

Jackie Aguas, IBCLC

Mariana Achugar, Ph.D., Carnegie Mellon University

Scott Rex, Ph.D., Southern Oregon University

Norma Lopez-Burton, M.A., University of California, Davis

■ ■ ■

WE ALSO GRATEFULLY ACKNOWLEDGE
THE FOLLOWING READERS
OF THE AUDIO PORTION OF THIS BOOK

Dulce Christensen

Leticia Martínez

Norma Sepúlveda

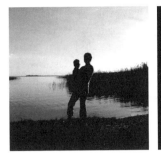

INTRODUCTION

WHY LEARN SPANISH FOR BREASTFEEDING SUPPORT?

As someone who works in breastfeeding support, you are committed to helping mothers breastfeed.

You know that communication is a critical element of your work. You've probably experienced the frustration of being unable to effectively communicate with mothers because of language barriers. You know you could be more effective with Spanish-speaking mothers if you had the right language skills.

This book is written for you – for the thousands of nurses, lactation consultants, WIC breastfeeding peer counselors, doctors, La Leche League leaders, midwives, childbirth educators, and others who help make breastfeeding work for families.

The need for Spanish language skills in medical settings is already great and is expected to grow in coming years. The Latino community in the U.S. is the fastest growing segment of our population. Between 2000 and 2050, the Latino population in the U.S. is projected to increase by 188 percent. By 2050, nearly one in four residents will be of Latino descent (U.S. Census Bureau, 2004). While not all Latinos speak Spanish as their primary language, many do.

In spite of this growth, Latinos are the most underrepresented ethnic group among registered nurses relative to their percentage of the population (Spartley et al., 2000). As the population of Spanish-speaking families grows, being able to communicate in Spanish becomes more and more important.

Latina mothers initiate breastfeeding at rates higher than the national average (Centers for Disease Control, n.d.). But research shows that mothers who have limited English skills are particularly at risk for receiving poor breastfeeding care (Feldman-Winter, 2004). They are less likely to receive basic breastfeeding care and to benefit from breastfeeding services, such as lactation support, assessments, and care plans--practices that are correlated to and predictive of exclusive breastfeeding. A recent study concluded, "Mothers with limited English proficiency represent a vulnerable population in the delivery hospital environment and warrant enhanced efforts to support exclusive breastfeeding" (Feldman-Winter, 2004).

ABOUT SPANISH FOR BREASTFEEDING SUPPORT

The goal of *Spanish for Breastfeeding Support* is to promote and support breastfeeding by giving you the tools you need to be effective with Spanish-speaking families.

Spanish for Breastfeeding Support can be used in four ways:

1) **AS A SELF-GUIDED COURSE.** This book is a complete self-guided course to learning Spanish to help breastfeeding mothers. The chapters provide dialogues on common breastfeeding topics, simple explanations of grammar, exercises with answers for self-evaluation, audio files to enhance listening and pronunciation, and "tear-out" sheets for quick reference.

2) **AS A TEXTBOOK IN A CLASSROOM SETTING.** This book can be used as a textbook in a Medical Spanish course designed for breastfeeding support professionals. Such a course could be held, for example, for the staff of a hospital's childbirth center or the staff of a WIC program. Each chapter includes teaching guidance for instructors presenting this material in a classroom setting.

3) **AS A REFERENCE BOOK.** This book can be used as a reference for situations requiring breastfeeding-related Spanish phrases, vocabulary, and other Spanish-language resources. A hospital or WIC office could make this book available to staff for use when needed.

4) **FOR CERPS.** International Board Certified Lactation Consultants can earn 12.8 continuing education recognition points (CERPs) for completing the exercises in this book.

The breastfeeding content in this book targets the most commonly discussed breastfeeding topics, such as latch and positioning, milk supply, and feeding frequency. Commonly used vocabulary, concepts, and expressions are taught as part of dialogues between mothers and breastfeeding support people. The dialogues are situated in a variety of settings, including hospital inpatient and outpatient settings, a pediatrician's office, a WIC office, and a breastfeeding support group meeting. The content also covers different stages in breastfeeding support, from early breastfeeding management through the return to work, the introduction of solid foods, and weaning.

It's easiest to learn a new language when you study it in a context that is interesting to you (Krashen, 2004), so the grammar and vocabulary in this book are always presented in the context of breastfeeding support. The lessons are tailored specifically to address the situations in which you encounter Spanish-speaking women and their families.

MATERIALS INCLUDED IN THIS BOOK

Spanish for Breastfeeding Support provides several resources to help you learn Spanish, including:

- Online MP3 files containing spoken versions of the dialogues presented in each chapter, as well as review conversations, vocabulary, pronunciation, listening exercises, and answers to exercises. See www.ibreastfeeding.com/SBFS.html to download audio files. Instructions are on the website.

- Illustrations that identify key vocabulary.

- Quick reference tear-out sheets at the end of each chapter listing key vocabulary and phrases.

- English-Spanish and Spanish-English glossaries of commonly used terms.

- A resource list of Spanish language publications, including patient print materials, bilingual helplines, web-based resources, and translated books and videos.

ADDITIONAL SUPPORT AVAILABLE ONLINE

Do you have questions or want additional exercises for practice? We've established a website to provide additional support and resources!

Visit www.spanishforbreastfeedingsupport.com for additional materials, links to patient handouts and CERP forms, and many other resources.

CERPS FOR INTERNATIONAL BOARD CERTIFIED LACTATION CONSULTANTS

Each chapter of this book has been approved as an independent study module. International Board Certified Lactation Consultants may earn CERPs for completing these modules. CERP forms are provided at the end of this book and on the website: www.spanishforbreastfeedingsupport.com.

To earn CERPs for completing some or all of the chapters in this book, fill out the CERP forms found in the appendix of this book, including:

- Answer sheet

- Self-directed evaluation

- Self-assessment questionnaire (complete only one if submitting several chapters)

You will need to complete CERP forms for each chapter for which you are requesting CERPs. Send these forms, along with payment for processing, to: Hale Publishing, 1712 N. Forest Street, Amarillo, TX 79106.

ADDITIONAL NOTES ON MEDICAL TRANSLATION AND SPANISH ACCENTS

This book is intended to help providers better communicate with Spanish-speaking mothers about basic breastfeeding management. It is not intended as a substitute for medical translation services, which can be critical in the delivery of medical care. This book is also not intended to substitute for efforts to create a more linguistically and culturally diverse workforce in the healthcare professions.

The Latino community in the U.S. is very diverse. There are many different Spanish accents spoken in this country. The Spanish on the accompanying audio files were recorded by Spanish speakers of Mexican descent. While this accent does not represent all Spanish speakers in the U.S., it was chosen because it represents the largest subgroup of Spanish speakers in the country. Please be aware that accent and expressions can vary by community and by region.

DIVERSE PRACTICES IN BREASTFEEDING SUPPORT

In this book, we have introduced a broad range of vocabulary and phrases, which may include terms that you don't use in your individual practice. For example, we mention herbs to increase milk supply in Chapter 5, but you may not use herbs in your practice. In Chapter 11, we discuss starting complementary foods with a tablespoon of solid food, but you may encourage mothers to allow babies to start with as much they want. We know that we cannot reflect all of the practices people use in breastfeeding support; our goal is to provide the widest possible range of vocabulary to help you help mothers. We hope that you will use what is useful to you.

CULTURE AND BREASTFEEDING

To be effective in supporting breastfeeding, it is critical to be knowledgeable about and respectful of mothers' cultural backgrounds. One way of demonstrating respect for a mother's culture is to attempt to communicate in her language. But this is not enough. How else can you show respect for mothers' cultural backgrounds?

- **ASK.** Ask mothers open-ended questions about their cultural traditions. We model this in Chapter 8. You'll both demonstrate respect and gain mothers' trust, and you will enrich your understanding of breastfeeding and mothering.

- **DON'T ASSUME.** Spanish-speaking mothers in the U.S. come from diverse cultural backgrounds, and there are regional and generational differences. It's important not to assume that you know what a mother believes or which traditions she follows. For example, don't assume that all Latina mothers speak Spanish fluently, or at all.

- **DON'T DISCOURAGE.** Don't discourage a cultural practice unless you believe it poses a health or safety risk. If a mother's culture dictates that she not eat pork during lactation, for example, there is no reason to discourage this practice.

- **EXPLAIN.** If there is a health concern, explain with sensitivity and respect why a particular tradition (not feeding colostrum, for example) is not in the health interest of the baby.

- **LEARN.** Take time to learn about cultural practices by asking mothers questions, reading about their cultures, and even participating in community events.

- **MAKE CHANGES.** As you learn more about different cultures in your community, work to make your hospital or office welcoming to mothers of all backgrounds. At one hospital, simply training staff and changing the menu offered to Cambodian mothers to reflect traditional dietary practices in the postpartum period increased breastfeeding initiation rates from 16% to 66% (Galvin et al., 2008).

A NOTE FROM THE SPANISH TEACHER

Learning a new language as an adult can be a challenging and rewarding endeavor. Just as you support women who may face challenges with breastfeeding, this book has been designed to be a source of support for you. Our hope is that this book will inspire you with a love of the Spanish language and help you to communicate more effectively with women and their families about breastfeeding.

To that end, here are some quick recommendations about being a self-taught language student:

- Be patient with yourself. It may take some time before you feel that you are communicating well with mothers. But with some practice, you'll soon be talking away!

- Practice is the key to success. Try to use the language as much as possible, both on the job and in your personal life. Visit www.spanishforbreastfeedingsupport.com for additional exercises and other resources.

- Use other media, including the resources in the back of this book, to increase your exposure to spoken and written Spanish (radio, television, magazines, websites).

- "You'll get out of it what you put into it." The more conscientious you are about listening to the audio and completing the exercises in the book, the more skills you will acquire and the more you will be able to communicate with mothers in Spanish.

- Strive not for perfection but for communication. We often make grammatical errors in our first language, yet we manage to communicate with one another. No one expects your spoken Spanish to be perfect. You may be surprised at how far your efforts to understand and speak some basic words and phrases will go toward gaining the trust and respect of your Spanish-speaking patients. And, trust and respect are the foundation of effective communication.

- Go for it! While you may feel shy at first, most mothers will be thrilled that you are making an effort to speak to them in a language that is more comfortable for them.

We wish you the very best!

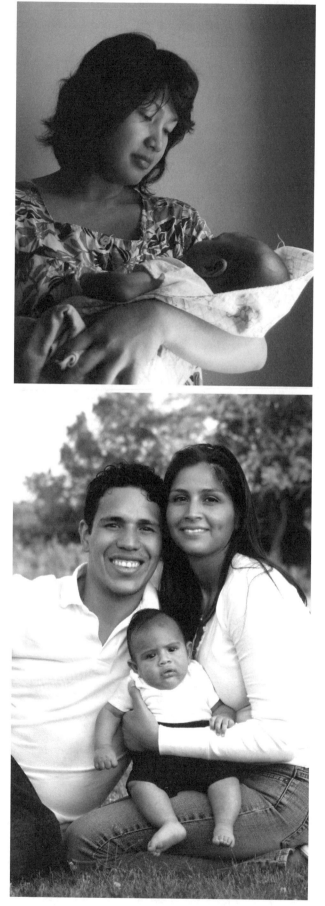

INTRODUCTORY ANATOMY

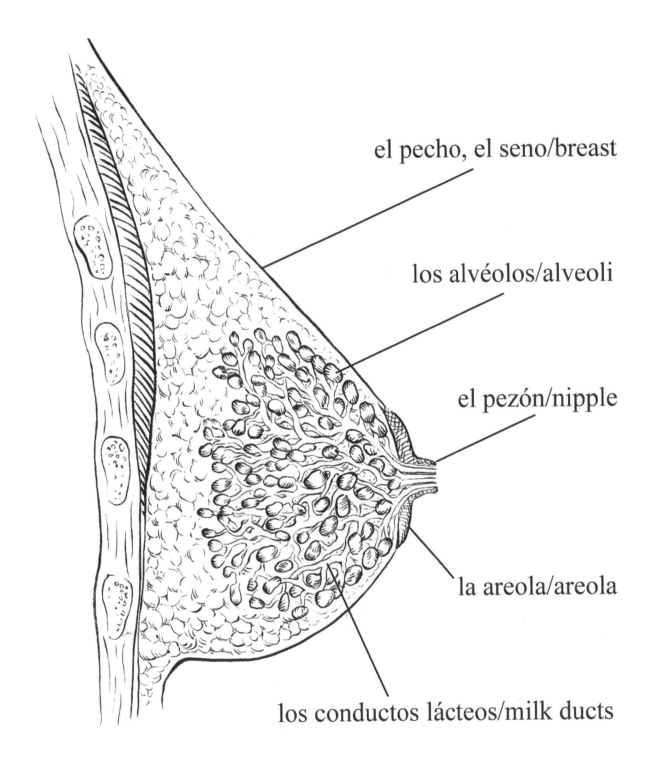

el pecho, el seno/breast

los alvéolos/alveoli

el pezón/nipple

la areola/areola

los conductos lácteos/milk ducts

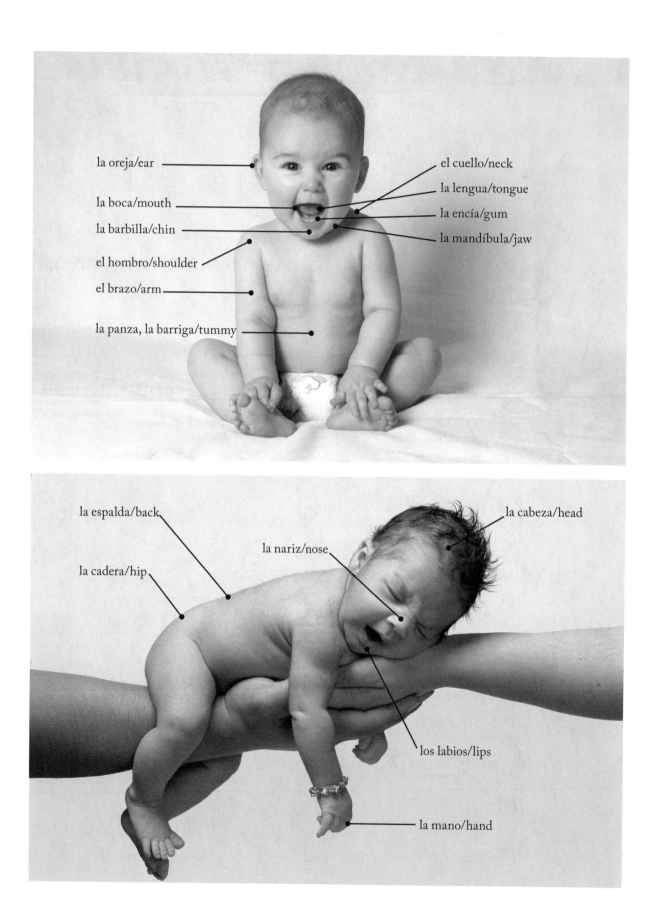

la oreja/ear

el cuello/neck

la lengua/tongue

la boca/mouth

la encía/gum

la barbilla/chin

la mandíbula/jaw

el hombro/shoulder

el brazo/arm

la panza, la barriga/tummy

la espalda/back

la cabeza/head

la nariz/nose

la cadera/hip

los labios/lips

la mano/hand

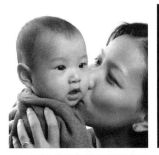

CHAPTER 1
BASIC GREETINGS AND CONVERSATION

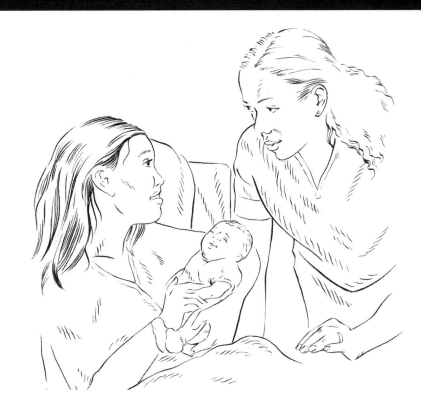

OBJECTIVES

By the end of
this chapter, you
will be able to:

• Understand and
use vocabulary and
phrases related to the
baby and the breast

• Pronounce the
sounds of the
Spanish alphabet

• Talk about people
and things

• Count from
one to 31

🎧 DIALOGUE

In this dialogue, a mother with a one-day-old baby and a nurse introduce themselves and begin talking about breastfeeding in the mother's hospital room. Listen to the dialogue as you read along in the book. Repeat each line, pausing the audio as necessary; then listen to the vocabulary and important phrases, and repeat each one.

Setting:
• **Postpartum hospital room**

Characters:
• **Nurse (Julie)**
• **Mother (Marta)**
• **One-day-old baby**

Nurse: Buenos días. Me llamo Julie. Soy su enfermera hoy.
[Good morning. My name is Julie. I'm your nurse for today.]

Mother: Hola. Mucho gusto. Me llamo Marta.
[Hi. Nice to meet you. My name is Marta.]

Nurse: Mucho gusto, Marta. Y, ¿cómo se llama su bebé?
[Nice to meet you, Marta. And what is your baby's name?]

Mother: Se llama José Ramón.
[His name is José Ramón.]

Nurse: Y, ¿cómo está usted?
[And, how are you?]

Mother: Estoy bien, pero cansada.
[I'm fine, but tired.]

Nurse: Sí, entiendo. ¿Cómo le va con la lactancia hoy?
[Yes, I understand. How is breastfeeding going today?]

Mother: Bueno, me preocupa que el bebé no reciba suficiente leche.
[Well, I'm worried that the baby isn't getting enough milk.]

Nurse: Lo siento, no entiendo. ¿Puede repetirlo otra vez más despacio, por favor? Sólo hablo un poco de español.
[I'm sorry, I don't understand. Would you say that again slowly, please? I only speak a little Spanish.]

Mother: Me preocupa que el bebé no reciba suficiente leche.
[I'm worried that the baby isn't getting enough milk.]

Nurse: O, entiendo, pero no se preocupe. Su cuerpo produce la cantidad perfecta de calostro para su bebé. Su estómago es muy pequeño ahora. Es sólo del tamaño de una…¿cómo se dice esto? (holding up a marble)
[Oh, I understand, but don't worry. Your body is producing the perfect amount of colostrum for your baby. His tummy is very small now. It's only as big as…how do you say this?] (holding up a marble)

Mother: Canica.
[Marble.]

Nurse: O, ¡gracias!
[Oh, thank you!]

Mother: ¿El calostro es buena leche?
[Is colostrum good milk?]

Nurse: Sí. El calostro es una leche especial que es muy buena para el bebé. Lo llamamos el "oro líquido."
[Yes. Colostrum is a special milk that is very good for your baby. We call it "liquid gold."]

Mother: Ya veo.
[I see.]

Nurse: ¿Desea ver su leche? Puedo enseñarle cómo extraer un poco de leche a mano.
[Would you like to see your milk? I can show you how to hand express some.]

Mother: Sí, por favor.
[Yes, please.]

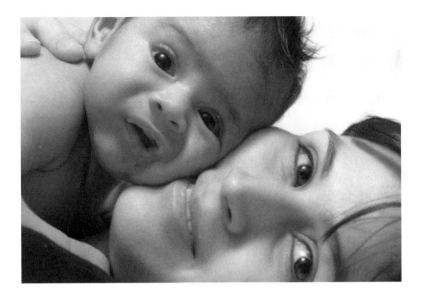

IMPORTANT PHRASES

1. Buenos días..Good morning.

2. Buenas tardes ....Good afternoon.

3. Buenas noches ....Good evening.

4. Soy su enfermera hoy .... I'm your nurse for today.

5. ¿Cómo está usted? ....How are you?

6. ¿Cómo se dice esto?..How do you say this?

7. ¿Cómo se llama?... What is your name?

8. Estoy bien...I'm fine.

9. Me llamo_____ ....My name is_____.

10. Mucho gusto .... Nice to meet you.

11. ¿Cómo le va con la lactancia? .... How is breastfeeding going?

12. Lo siento ....I'm sorry.

13. No entiendo.. I don't understand.

14. ¿Puede repetirlo otra vez   Would you say that again
    más despacio, por favor? .... slowly, please?

15. Sólo hablo un   I only speak
    poco de español... a little Spanish.

16. No se preocupe .... Don't worry.

17. Extraer la leche a mano .... to hand express, to manually express

18. Ya veo ....I see.

COMPREHENSION QUESTIONS

Exercise 1. After reading and listening to the dialogue on the audio file, listen again without the text and answer the following questions. Try to answer question 2 in Spanish.

Note: If you are completing the exercises in this chapter for CERPs, write your answers on the answer sheet provided in Appendix A.

1. What is the name of Marta's baby?

El bebé se llama...

a. Alejandro

b. José Ramón

c. Javier

d. Juan José

2. What is Marta worried about?

Marta se preocupa que su bebé...

_____

3. What does the nurse tell Marta about colostrum?

El calostro es...

a. una leche especial

b. muy buena para el bebé

c. el "oro líquido"

d. all of the above

🎧 LANGUAGE LESSONS

Introductory Anatomy. Listen to the speaker read the anatomy terms as you study the illustrations of the baby and the breast, and practice repeating each term.

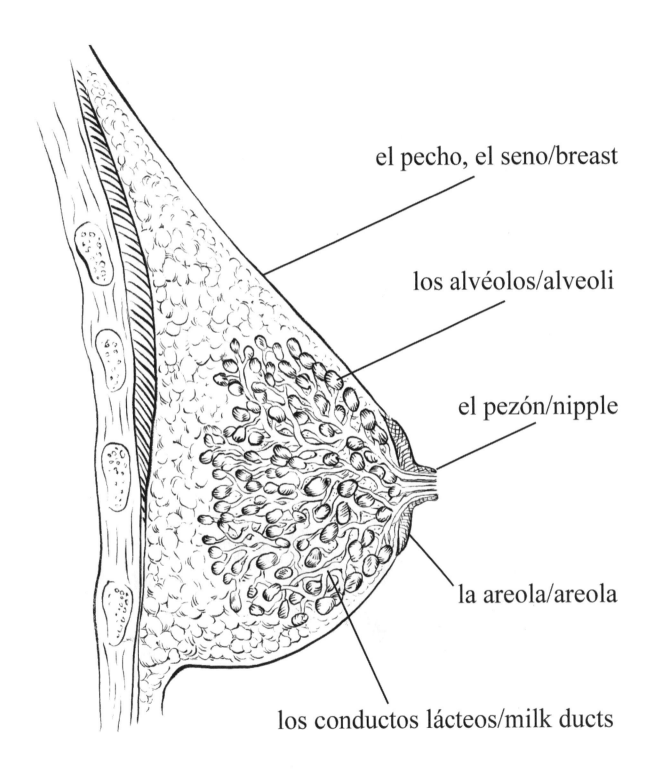

el pecho, el seno/breast

los alvéolos/alveoli

el pezón/nipple

la areola/areola

los conductos lácteos/milk ducts

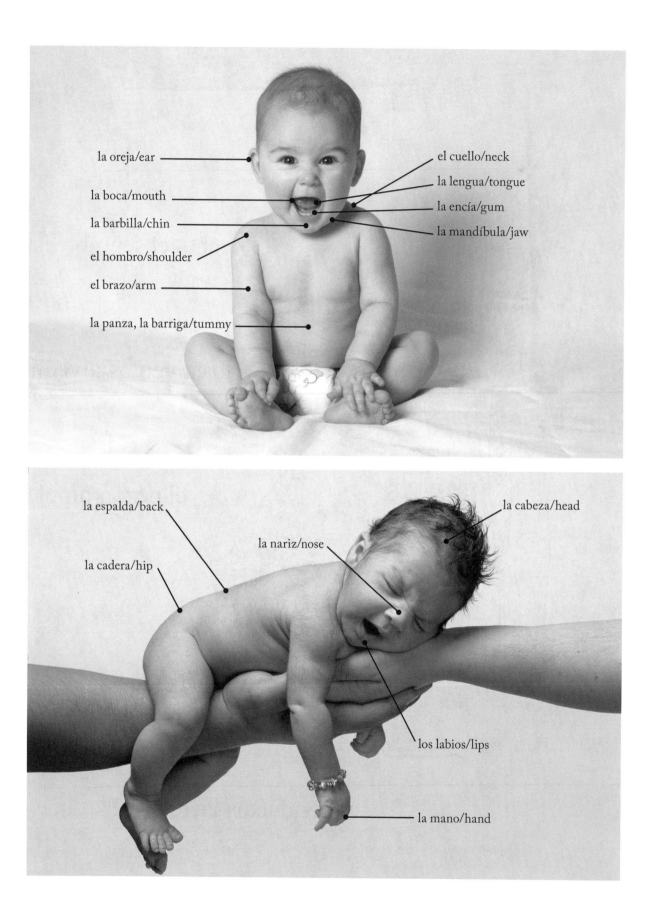

la oreja/ear

la boca/mouth

la barbilla/chin

el hombro/shoulder

el brazo/arm

la panza, la barriga/tummy

el cuello/neck

la lengua/tongue

la encía/gum

la mandíbula/jaw

la espalda/back

la cadera/hip

la nariz/nose

la cabeza/head

los labios/lips

la mano/hand

🎧 A. THE SPANISH ALPHABET

The pronunciation of Spanish is simple because of its consistency. Unlike the English language, the sounds of Spanish vowels are always the same, even in combination with each other. Listen to the speaker read the Spanish alphabet, vowels, and consonants, and practice repeating each sound.

a	a	**n**	ene
b	be	**ñ**	eñe
c	ce	**o**	o
d	de	**p**	pe
e	e	**q**	cu
f	efe	**r**	ere
g	ge	**s**	ese
h	hache	**t**	te
i	i	**u**	u
j	jota	**v**	ve
k	ka	**w**	doble v
l	ele	**x**	equis
ll	elle	**y**	i griega
m	eme	**z**	zeta

Vowels:

a (ā) as in "saw"

e (ā) as in "gray"

i (ē) as in "see"

o (ō) as in "snow"

u (ōō) as in "food"

Consonants:

ll (y sound)

ñ (nya)

r (short roll)

rr (long roll)

✎ **Exercise 2.** Listen to the speaker read a series of letters in Spanish, and write each letter down to spell the vocabulary word from this chapter.

1. ___ ___ ___ ___

2. ___ ___ ___ ___ ___

3. ___ ___ ___ ___ ___ ___

4. ___ ___ ___ ___ ___ ___

5. ___ ___ ___ ___ ___

Note: Emphasis and Accents. There are three basic rules for determining where to place the emphasis when pronouncing a word in Spanish.

1. All words ending in n, s, or a vowel carry the stress on the second to last syllable of the word.
   Examples: espalda: esPALda
            conductos: conDUCTos

2. Words ending with any other letter carry the stress on the last syllable.
   Examples: nariz: naRIZ
            cantidad: cantiDAD

3. When a word has an accent, the stress goes on the syllable carrying the accent mark. The presence of an accent mark overrides Rules 1 and 2.
   Examples: pezón: peZÓN
            mandíbula: manDÍbula

B. TALKING ABOUT PEOPLE AND THINGS

The Spanish language assigns every person and thing a "gender," either masculine or feminine. When talking about people, the gender is obvious. When talking about things, the designation of "masculine" or "feminine" has nothing to do with the object itself, but depends on the spelling of the word (with a few important exceptions). In general, most words ending in "o" are masculine, while most words ending in "a" are feminine.

It is much more common to use "the" in front of a noun in Spanish than it is in English. You'll notice that in the introductory anatomy, each item was preceded by *"el"* (masculine) or *"la"* (feminine), or sometimes *"los"* (more than one masculine noun) or *"las"* (more than one feminine noun).

Note: When referring to both masculine and feminine objects together, the masculine is used. For example, a group of boy and girl children is referred to as *"los niños."*

Gender is important in two situations: first, when we want to say "the" or "a/an" in front of the word, and second, when using an adjective to describe a person or thing (discussed in Chapter 4).

"THE" IN SPANISH: EL, LA, LOS, LAS	
El pecho *[the breast]*	Los pechos *[the breasts]*
El pezón *[the nipple]*	Los pezones *[the nipples]*
La boca *[the mouth]*	Las bocas *[the mouths]*
La lengua *[the tongue]*	Las lenguas *[the tongues]*

"A" OR "AN" OR "SOME" IN SPANISH: UN, UNA, UNOS, UNAS	
Un bebé *[a baby]*	Unos bebés *[some babies]*
Un seno *[a breast]*	Unos senos *[some breasts]*
Una enfermera *[a nurse]*	Unas enfermeras *[some nurses]*
Una madre *[a mother]*	Unas madres *[some mothers]*

When learning to speak Spanish, it's natural to confuse the gender of words. While gender is an important aspect of understanding spoken Spanish, you can still communicate well, even if you struggle with this system.

Exercise 3. Indicate the word for "the" in front of each person or thing.

1. _____ areola

2. _____ cabeza

3. _____ pezón

4. _____ labios

5. _____ enfermeras

Exercise 4. Indicate the word for "a," "an," or "some" in front of each person or thing.

1. _____ madre

2. _____ pecho

3. _____ lengua

4. _____ alvéolos

5. _____ doctoras

Exercise 5. Use the glossary at the end of this book to look up the gender of the following words. Each noun is followed by "m" or "f" to indicate masculine or feminine. Look for exceptions to the basic rules you have learned. In the second column, indicate whether the noun in the first column is masculine or feminine. In the third column, write the Spanish word for "the" in front of each noun.

Glossary Term	Gender (m or f)	"The"
1. Pezón		_____ pezón
2. Nariz		_____ nariz
3. Mano		_____ mano
4. Calostro		_____ calostro
5. Problema		_____ problema
6. Familia		_____ familia
7. Alergia		_____ alergia
8. Pañal		_____ pañal
9. Padre		_____ padre
10. Piel		_____ piel

C. NUMBERS 1-31

Listen to the speaker read the numbers from 1 to 31, and repeat each one.

1: uno	9: nueve	17: diecisiete	25: veinticinco
2: dos	10: diez	18: dieciocho	26: veintiséis
3: tres	11: once	19: diecinueve	27: veintisiete
4: cuatro	12: doce	20: veinte	28: veintiocho
5: cinco	13: trece	21: veintiuno	29: veintinueve
6: seis	14: catorce	22: veintidós	30: treinta
7: siete	15: quince	23: veintitrés	31: treinta y uno
8: ocho	16: dieciséis	24: veinticuatro	

Exercise 6. Listen as the speaker reads 15 numbers in Spanish; then write the numbers in the spaces below.

1. _____   6. _____   11. _____

2. _____   7. _____   12. _____

3. _____   8. _____   13. _____

4. _____   9. _____   14. _____

5. _____   10. _____   15. _____

LISTENING COMPREHENSION

Exercise 7. Listen to the dialogue on the audio file between a nurse and the mother of a newborn as they discuss breastfeeding; then answer the comprehension questions in English.

1.   What is the nurse's name?

     _____

2.   What is the baby's name?

     _____

3.   How does Elena feel today?

     _____

4.   What does Elena want to know about colostrum?

     _____

5.   What does the nurse call colostrum?

     _____

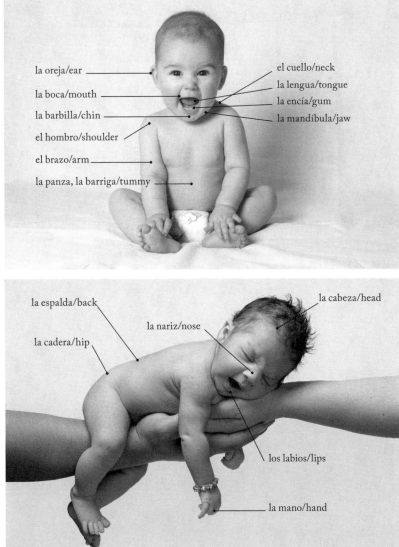

la oreja/ear
el cuello/neck
la lengua/tongue
la boca/mouth
la encía/gum
la barbilla/chin
la mandíbula/jaw
el hombro/shoulder
el brazo/arm
la panza, la barriga/tummy

la espalda/back
la cabeza/head
la nariz/nose
la cadera/hip
los labios/lips
la mano/hand

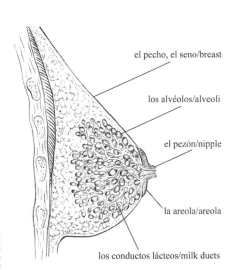

el pecho, el seno/breast

los alvéolos/alveoli

el pezón/nipple

la areola/areola

los conductos lácteos/milk ducts

COMMON GREETINGS AND STATEMENTS

Good morning.
Buenos días.

Good afternoon.
Buenas tardes.

Good evening.
Buenas noches.

My name is …
Me llamo …

What is your name?
¿Cómo se llama?

Nice to meet you.
Mucho gusto.

Can you repeat that, please?
¿Puede repetirlo, por favor?

How is breastfeeding going?
¿Cómo le va con la lactancia?

How are you?
¿Cómo está usted?

How do you say this?
¿Cómo se dice esto?

I only speak a little Spanish.
Sólo hablo un poco de español.

I am fine.
Estoy bien.

I'm sorry, I don't understand.
Lo siento, no entiendo.

Don't worry.
No se preocupe.

NOTES FOR THE CLASSROOM INSTRUCTOR

This section is for instructors using this book in a classroom setting.

Much of the work in this beginning chapter must be done by the student. The most important role for the teacher is to lower the students' affective filter and make sure that their focus remains on understanding the key terms they will use and becoming comfortable with pronunciation. Some suggested activities include:

SECTION A: ALPHABET

1. Have students give each other "eye exams" (ask them to read individual letters from a chart).

2. Working in pairs, have students spell their names for each other.

3. As an interactive game with the class, spell vocabulary words out loud, saying each letter slowly. Award a prize to the first student who guesses what word you are spelling and shouts it out to the group. The winner finishes spelling the word for the class.

SECTION C: NUMBERS

1. Provide simple math problems for the students to write in Spanish. For example:

Q: 3 x 5 = ?

A: tres por cinco son quince

2. Have students circulate throughout the room asking for phone numbers of other students in Spanish and writing them down on a piece of paper.

BASIC CONVERSATION

1. Start each class with a warm-up activity, such as asking, "How do you feel?" questions, telling a joke of the day, and/or doing activities with vocabulary words to be introduced during that class period.

2. Divide students into pairs and ask them to write short dialogues to present in front of the class, using the vocabulary in the chapter.

ANSWER KEY

Need help with these exercises? Looking for more opportunities to practice? For support and additional resources to help you learn to provide breastfeeding support in Spanish, visit www.spanishforbreastfeedingsupport.com.

Exercise 1.

1. b. José Ramón

2. no reciba suficiente leche

3. d. all of the above

Exercise 2.

1. boca

2. pezón

3. areola

4. labios

5. pecho

Exercise 3.

1. la

2. la

3. el

4. los

5. las

Exercise 4.

1. una

2. un

3. una

4. unos

5. unas

Exercise 5.

1. Pezón: m., el pezón

2. Nariz: f., la nariz

3. Mano: f., la mano

4. Calostro: m., el calostro

5. Problema: m., el problema

6. Familia: f., la familia

7. Alergia: f., la alergia

8. Pañal: m., el pañal

9. Padre: m., el padre

10. Piel: f., la piel

Exercise 6.

1. 10

2. 7

3. 14

4. 23

5. 5

6. 11

7. 12

8. 30

9. 3

10. 19

11. 15

12. 20

13. 8

14. 29

15. 16

Listening Comprehension Dialogue

Nurse: ¡Buenos días! Me llamo Julie, soy su enfermera hoy.

[Good morning! My name is Julie, I'm your nurse for today.]

Mother: Hola, me llamo Elena y mi bebé se llama Nicolas.

[Hi, I'm Elena, and my baby's name is Nicolas.]

Nurse: ¿Cómo está hoy?

[How are you today?]

Mother: Estoy bien, pero cansada.

[I'm fine, but tired.]

Nurse: Sí, entiendo. Y, ¿cómo le va con la lactancia?

[Yes, I understand. And how is breastfeeding going?]

Mother: Bueno, me preocupa que el bebé no reciba suficiente leche.

[Well, I'm worried that the baby isn't getting enough milk.]

Nurse: Su bebé recibe el calostro y su estómago es muy pequeño ahora.

[Your baby is getting your colostrum, and his tummy is very small now.]

Mother: ¿El calostro es buena leche?

[Is the colostrum good milk?]

Nurse: Sí, es una leche muy especial. Lo llamamos el oro líquido.

[Yes, it's a very special milk. We call it liquid gold.]

Exercise 7.

1. Julie

2. Nicolas

3. She's fine, but tired.

4. Is it good milk?

5. "liquid gold"

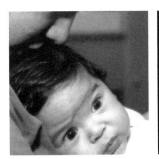

CHAPTER 2
POSITIONING

OBJECTIVES

By the end of
this chapter, you
will be able to:

• Understand and
use vocabulary and
phrases related
to positioning

• Refer to people
and things

• Use basic
action words

• Understand and use
days of the week and
months of the year

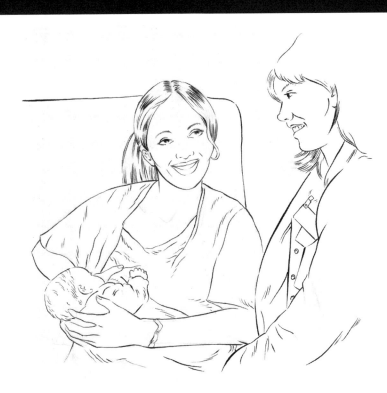

🎧 DIALOGUE

In this dialogue, a nurse and a mother of a two-day-old baby are discussing positioning in the mother's hospital room. Listen to the dialogue as you read along in the book. Repeat each line, pausing the audio as necessary; then listen to the vocabulary and important phrases, and repeat each one.

Setting:
• **Postpartum hospital room**

Characters:
• **Nurse (Karen)**
• **Mother (Angela)**
• **2-day-old baby**

Nurse: Buenos días, Angela. ¿Cómo puedo ayudarla hoy?
[Good morning, Angela. How can I help you today?]

Mother: No sé cómo sostener al bebé cuando le doy pecho. ¿Me puede ayudar con eso?
[I don't know how to hold the baby when I breastfeed him. Can you help me with that?]

Nurse: Sí. Comencemos con el bebé piel con piel contra su pecho.
[Sure. Let's start with your baby skin-to-skin on your chest.]

Mother: ¿Qué significa "piel con piel"?
[What's skin-to-skin?]

Nurse: Bueno, el bebé lleva solo el pañal y descansa sobre su pecho descubierto entre los senos.
[Well, the baby wears only his diaper and lies on your bare chest between your breasts.]

Mother: ¿Así?
[Like this?]

Nurse: Sí, ¡Excelente! ¿Puede ver que busca el pecho?
[Yes, that's great! Do you see him looking for the breast?]

Mother: Sí. ¿Ahora qué hago?
[Yes. What do I do now?]

Nurse: Ponga las manos en su espalda y hombros y ayúdele a ponerse "panza con panza." Sosténgalo muy cerca de usted.
[Put your hands on his back and shoulders, and help him get "tummy to tummy." Hold him very close to you.]

Mother: ¿Así?
[Like this?]

Nurse: ¡Sí, muy bien! Su oreja, hombro y cadera deben estar en una línea recta y debe estar "nariz contra el pezón."
[Yes, very good! His ear, shoulder, and hip should be in a straight line, and he should be "nose to nipple."]

Mother: OK
[Okay]

Nurse: Y sostenga el pecho con la otra mano.
[And hold your breast with your other hand.]

Mother: ¿Así?
[Like this?]

Nurse: ¡Muy bien! Esta posición se llama la posición de cuna cruzada. Ahora vamos a ayudar al bebé a pegarse al pecho. Más tarde le enseño la posición de lado y la posición acostada.
[Very good! This position is called the cross-cradle hold. Next, we'll help him get latched on. Later, I'll show you the football hold and the side lying hold.]

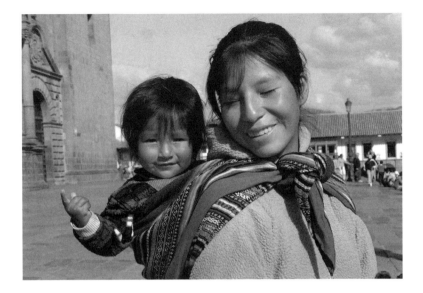

IMPORTANT PHRASES

1. Me va bien...It's going well for me.

2. Bueno ....Well.

3. ¿Cómo puedo ayudarla? ....How can I help you?

4. Comencemos con el bebé piel   Let's start with the baby
con piel contra su pecho..............................skin-to-skin on your chest.

5. No sé ....I don't know.

6. ¿Qué significa ____? .... What does ____ mean?

7. ¡Muy bien!.. Very good!

8. ¡Muy bien hecho!...Good job, well done.

9. Así .... Like this.

COMPREHENSION QUESTIONS

Exercise 1. After reading and listening to the dialogue on the audio file, listen again without the text and answer the following questions.

Note: If you are completing the exercises in this chapter for CERPs, write your answers on the answer sheets provided in Appendix A.

  1. What does Angela say she needs help with?
     No sé cómo...

     a. alimentar al bebé

     b. sostener al bebé

     c. cambiar el pañal del bebé

     d. encontrar una posición cómoda

2. How does the nurse say that Angela and her baby should begin?

    a. en la cama

    b. acostados

    c. piel con piel contra su pecho

    d. en el hospital

3. How should the baby be positioned to begin breastfeeding?

    a. panza con panza

    b. nariz contra el pezón

    c. oreja, hombro, cadera en una línea recta

    d. all of the above

4. Where should Angela position her hands?

    a. una mano en la espalda y los hombros del bebé y otra en su seno

    b. una mano en la panza y otra en el pecho del bebé

    c. una mano en la espalda y otra en el cuello del bebé

    d. una mano en la cabeza y otra en el brazo del bebé

5. What position does the nurse help Angela get into?

    a. posición acostada

    b. posición de cuna cruzada

    c. posición de lado

    d. posición sandía

LANGUAGE LESSONS

A. REFERRING TO PEOPLE AND THINGS

Often, we use noun substitutes (pronouns) like "she," "he," "it," and "they" to refer to people or things. In Spanish, these words are:

Yo	I	Nosotros	We (masculine)
Tú	You (informal)	Nosotras	We (feminine)
Usted/Ustedes	You (formal)	Ellos	They (masculine)
Él, Ella, Él	He, She, It	Ellas	They (feminine)

Examples:

• Ella pone al bebé panza con panza. *[She places the baby tummy to tummy.]*

• Nosotros podemos ayudarla con la posición del bebé. *[We can help you position the baby.]*

• Él debe estar nariz contra el pezón. *[He should be nose to nipple.]*

Note: When speaking in Spanish, demonstrating respect toward others is very important. There are two ways to say "you" when speaking directly to another person. The first of these is the informal *tú*, which is used with children, friends, and people who are close to you, such as close family members. The formal *usted* is used when speaking with unknown people, those in positions of authority, or any situation in which you wish to demonstrate respect (for example, with one's elders). In a medical setting, it is most appropriate to use the formal *usted* to demonstrate respect for the patient.

Exercise 2. Find the appropriate pronoun to substitute for the person/s described in the following sentences.

Example: María has a baby.

> *Ella tiene un bebé.*

1. The baby's father can help with breastfeeding.

_____ puede ayudar con la lactancia.

2. The other lactation consultants and I sometimes recommend the football hold.

_____a veces recomendamos la posición sandía.

3. The mother is worried about her baby.

_____ está preocupada por su bebé.

4. Mothers sometimes do not know how to position the baby.

_____ a veces no saben cómo colocar al bebé.

5. Fathers also can ask the nurse for help.

_____también pueden pedirle ayuda a la enfermera.

6. I know you (formal) are worried about milk supply.

Sé que _____ está preocupada por la cantidad de leche que su cuerpo produce.

7. How are you all? (formal, plural)

¿Cómo están_____?

B. INTRODUCTION TO CONJUGATING VERBS

In Spanish, action words (verbs) are made up of a stem and an ending.

STEM	ENDING
Coloc	-ar
Colocar (to place)	

All verbs end in either *-ar*, *-er*, or *-ir*. For example:

Ayud**ar** = to help

Com**er** = to eat

Escrib**ir** = to write

When using a verb in a sentence, it must be conjugated according to the person taking the action described.

A verb is conjugated by removing the *-ar*, *-er*, or *-ir* ending and adding a different ending to the stem. Each "person" (I, you, he/she/it, we, they) has a corresponding ending. For example:

- Ella ayud**a** = she helps

- Nosotros ayud**amos** = we help

- Ellos ayud**an** = they help

Note: Because each person has a different ending, it is often not necessary to indicate the pronoun or person taking the action in front of the verb. For example:

- (Nosotras) ayudamos a las madres con la colocación de sus bebés.

[We help the mothers with positioning their babies.]

In this sentence, we can tell from the ending of the conjugated form of *ayudar* (–amos), that "we" is the subject of the verb; therefore, the inclusion of "*nosotras*" is not necessary.

Each of the three types of verbs (-*ar*, -*er*, -*ir*) has spelling rules for its endings, and there are several irregular verbs with special conjugations. These rules are different depending on whether you are describing something that is happening right now, in the future, or in the past. We will begin with the present tense to describe what's happening now.

C. Present Tense Conjugation

-AR VERBS		-ER VERBS		-IR VERBS	
Yo: **-o**	Nosotros: **-amos**	Yo: **-o**	Nosotros: **-emos**	Yo: **-o**	Nosotros: **-imos**
Tú: **-as**		Tú: **-es**		Tú: **-es**	
Él, Ella, Usted: **-a**	Ellos, Ustedes: **-an**	Él, Ella, Usted: **-e**	Ellos, Ustedes: **-en**	Él, Ella, Usted: **-e**	Ellos, Ustedes: **-en**

Ayudar (to help)		Comer (to eat)		Recibir (to receive)	
Yo: ayud**o**	Nosotros: ayud**amos**	Yo: com**o**	Nosotros: com**emos**	Yo: recib**o**	Nosotros: recib**imos**
Tú: ayud**as**		Tú: com**es**		Tú: recib**es**	
Él, Ella, Usted: ayud**a**	Ellos, Ustedes: ayud**an**	Él, Ella, Usted: com**e**	Ellos, Ustedes: com**en**	Él, Ella, Usted: recib**e**	Ellos, Ustedes: recib**en**

Exercise 3. Conjugate the –ar verb in the following sentences.

1. El bebé (descansar) _____ sobre el pecho descubierto de su mamá.
   [The baby rests on his mother's bare chest.]

2. Las mamás (acunar) _____ a los bebés para dar pecho.
   [Mothers cradle their babies in order to breastfeed.]

3. Nosotros (ayudar) _____ a las madres con la posición de sus bebés.
   [We help the mothers with the position of their babies.]

4. Yo (colocar) _____ a la bebé en la posición sandía.
   [I place the baby in the football hold.]

5. El bebé (llevar) _____ sólo el pañal.
   [The baby wears only a diaper.]

Exercise 4. Conjugate the –er and –ir verbs in the following sentences.

1. La bebé (comer) _____ cada dos horas aproximadamente.
   [The baby eats about every two hours.]

2. Nosotras (escribir) _____ las instrucciones para las madres.
   [We write the instructions for the mothers.]

3. Las enfermeras (aprender) _____ el español.
   [The nurses learn Spanish.]

4. La bebé (recibir) _____ suficiente leche.
   [The baby receives enough milk.]

5. Las madres (beber) _____ agua cuando tienen sed.
   [The mothers drink when they are thirsty.]

D. Common Irregular Conjugations in the Present Tense

There are some verbs that do not follow the rules. They are called irregular verbs. Irregular conjugations in the present tense come in three basic forms: those that are only different in the first-person *yo* form, those that require a different spelling of the stem, and the rest—those verbs that don't have easy rules, but must be memorized.

In this chapter and the next two, we will introduce some of the more common irregular present tense verbs that you will use in breastfeeding support, beginning with the following three examples:

DAR (TO GIVE)		TENER (TO HAVE)		PONER (TO PUT, TO PLACE)	
Yo: **doy**	Nosotros: **damos**	Yo: teng**o**	Nosotros: ten**emos**	Yo: pong**o**	Nosotros: pon**emos**
Tú: **das**		Tú: tien**es**		Tú: pon**es**	
Él, Ella, Usted: **da**	Ellos, Ustedes: **dan**	Él, Ella, Usted: tien**e**	Ellos, Ustedes: tien**en**	Él, Ella, Usted: pon**e**	Ellos, Ustedes: pon**en**

Examples:

- Yo doy una clase sobre la lactancia.
  [I give (teach) a class on breastfeeding.]

- Las madres tienen mucha leche.
  [Mothers have a lot of milk.]

- Pongo a mi bebé en la posición de cuna.
  [I place my baby in cradle hold.]

Exercise 5. Conjugate the irregular verbs in the following sentences.

1. Las enfermeras (dar) _____ clases sobre la lactancia.
   [The nurses give (teach) classes on breastfeeding.]

2. Marta (tener) _____ mucha leche.
   [Marta has a lot of milk.]

3. Yo (poner) _____ a la bebé en la posición acostada.
   [I place the baby in the side-lying hold.]

4. Usted (poner) _____ la mano en la espalda y los hombros del bebé.
   [You place your hand on the baby's back and shoulders.]

5. Yo (dar) _____ pecho cada dos horas.
   [I breastfeed every two hours.]

E. Days of the Week and Months of the Year

Listen to the speaker read the days of the week and the months of the year, and repeat each one. The days of the week are always masculine (*el, un*) and are not capitalized.

lunes: Monday	**viernes:** Friday
martes: Tuesday	**sábado:** Saturday
miércoles: Wednesday	**domingo:** Sunday
jueves: Thursday	

Months are not preceded by the word "the," but are considered masculine. Months also are not capitalized.

enero: January	**julio:** July
febrero: February	**agosto:** August
marzo: March	**septiembre:** September
abril: April	**octubre:** October
mayo: May	**noviembre:** November
junio: June	**diciembre:** December

F. PUTTING IT ALL TOGETHER: DATES

Now that you know some numbers, days, and months, you can say and understand dates. In Spanish, dates are given in the following way:

Tuesday, March 4 = martes, el cuatro de marzo

The only exception to this format is the first day of the month, which is written as "the first." For example, May 1ˢᵗ is written, *"el primero de mayo"* (the first of May).

Exercise 6. Practice writing the following dates in Spanish.

1. Monday, October 14

_____

2. Thursday, May 15

_____

3. Sunday, November 1

_____

4. Wednesday, June 18

_____

5. Tuesday, August 7

_____

Exercise 7. *¿Cuándo nació el bebé?* When was the baby born? Often in practice, you will need to ask mothers how old their babies are or when they were born. In this exercise, write the dates in Spanish to indicate when each baby was born.

Example: ¿Cuándo nació el bebé? (January 4)
      El cuatro de enero.

1. ¿Cuándo nació la bebé? (February 10)

_____

2. ¿Cuándo nació Alejandro? (March 9)

_____

3. ¿Cuándo nació Francisco? (December 22)

_____

4. ¿Cuándo nació el bebé? (June 27)

_____

5. ¿Cuándo nació Eva? (September 26)

_____

LANGUAGE REVIEW: INTRODUCTIONS AND GREETINGS

 Exercise 8. Match each question or statement with its corresponding response based on the greetings and exchanges that appeared in the Chapter 1 dialogues.

1. ¿Cómo se llama?   a. Mucho gusto.

2. Me llamo Melissa.   b. Me va bien, gracias.

3. ¿Cómo le va con la lactancia?   c. Estoy bien, pero cansada.

4. ¿Cómo está usted?   d. Me llamo Dalia.

LISTENING COMPREHENSION

Exercise 9. Listen to the dialogue on the audio file between a nurse and the mother of a newborn as they discuss positioning; then answer the comprehension questions in English.

1. What is the first thing the nurse suggests the mother do?

a. darle el calostro al bebé

b. sostener el pecho

c. poner al bebé piel con piel

d. poner al bebé panza con panza

2. What does the baby start to do?

a. buscar el pecho

b. descansar

c. comer

d. colocar

3. How does the mother hold the baby?

a. en la posición lateral

b. en la posición acostada

c. en la posición de cuna

d. panza con panza y nariz contra el pezón

TEAR-OUT QUICK REFERENCE: POSITIONING

KEY VOCABULARY	
ENGLISH	**SPANISH**
to hold	sostener
position, hold	posición
cradle hold	posición de cuna
cross cradle hold	posición de cuna cruzada
football hold	posición de lado, de fútbol americano, de sandía
side-lying hold	posición acostada
skin-to-skin	piel con piel
tummy-to-tummy	panza con panza
nose to nipple	nariz contra el pezón

DAYS OF THE WEEK	
ENGLISH	**SPANISH**
Monday	lunes
Tuesday	martes
Wednesday	miércoles
Thursday	jueves
Friday	viernes
Saturday	sábado
Sunday	domingo

MONTHS OF THE YEAR	
ENGLISH	**SPANISH**
January	enero
February	febrero
March	marzo
April	abril
May	mayo
June	junio
July	julio
August	agosto
September	septiembre
October	octubre
November	noviembre
December	diciembre

COMMON PHRASES	
ENGLISH	**SPANISH**
How can I help you?	¿Cómo puedo ayudarla?
Let's start with the baby skin-to-skin on your chest.	Comencemos con el bebé piel con piel contra su pecho.
Place the baby tummy-to-tummy.	Ponga al bebé "panza con panza."
The baby should be nose to nipple.	El bebé debe estar "nariz contra el pezón."

Notes for the Classroom Instructor

This section is for instructors using this book in a classroom setting.

Sections C and D: Present tense conjugation, regular and irregular verbs

1. Using verbs that have already been presented in Chapters 1 and 2, the teacher can create a sheet of 10-12 statements and ask the students to "interview" each other and identify students who agree with the statements (e.g., "Has children," "Eats Italian food," "Wears earrings.").

2. Because conjugation requires memorization, it may be helpful to provide additional worksheets with conjugation practice, particularly with irregular verbs. You can also encourage students to create their own conjugation flashcards for the most common words they will use on the job.

3. It is helpful to emphasize the importance of protocol and the use of *usted* in dealing with patients. Give students extra practice and reinforce proper greetings through speaking exercises in class.

Sections E and F: Days, Months, and Dates

1. There are several fun activities for the classroom involving days, months, and dates. If the size of the class allows (no more than about 15-20 students), you can ask the students to get into chronological order by birth date. This requires them to ask each other for their birthdays and organize themselves into a chronological line. If the class is larger, students can organize themselves according to birth month.

2. Note about abbreviation of dates: It is important for students who consult documents created in Latin America to understand that the Spanish formation of dates reverses the month and day from their order in English. For example, in English, 7/9/85 is July 9, 1985. In Spanish, that abbreviation would signify September 7, 1985. In other words, the order in Spanish is day, month, year.

ANSWER KEY

Need help with these exercises? Looking for more opportunities to practice? For support and additional resources to help you learn to provide breastfeeding support in Spanish, visit www.spanishforbreastfeedingsupport.com.

Exercise 1.

1. b
2. c
3. d
4. a
5. b

Exercise 2.

1. Él
2. Nosotros or Nosotras
3. Ella
4. Ellas
5. Ellos
6. usted
7. ustedes

Exercise 3.

1. descansa
2. acunan
3. ayudamos
4. coloco
5. lleva

Exercise 4.

1. come
2. escribimos
3. aprenden
4. recibe
5. beben

Exercise 5.

1. dan
2. tiene
3. pongo
4. pone
5. doy

Exercise 6.

1. lunes, el catorce de octubre
2. jueves, el quince de mayo
3. domingo, el primero de noviembre
4. miércoles, el dieciocho de junio
5. martes, el siete de agosto

Exercise 7.

1. el diez de febrero
2. el nueve de marzo
3. el veintidós de diciembre
4. el veintisiete de junio
5. el veintiséis de septiembre

Exercise 8.

1. d
2. a
3. b
4. c

Listening Comprehension Dialogue

Nurse: Vamos a poner al bebé piel con piel.

[Let's place your baby skin-to-skin.]

Mother: ¿Así?

[Like this?]

Nurse: Sí. ¿Ve que está buscando el pecho?
[Yes. Do you see him looking for the breast?]

Mother: ¡Sí! ¿Qué debo hacer ahora?
[Yes! What should I do now?]

Nurse: Vamos a ponerlo panza con panza.
[Let's place him tummy-to-tummy.]

Mother: ¿Así?

[Like this?]

Nurse: Sí, y debe estar nariz contra el pezón.
[Yes, and he should be positioned nose to nipple.]

Mother: Y, ¿debo sostener el pecho con la otra mano?
[And should I hold my breast with the other hand?]

Nurse: Sí. ¡Muy bien hecho!
[Yes. Great job!]

Exercise 9.

1. c
2. a
3. d

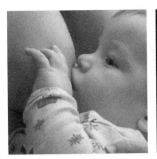

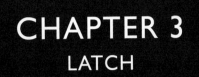

CHAPTER 3
LATCH

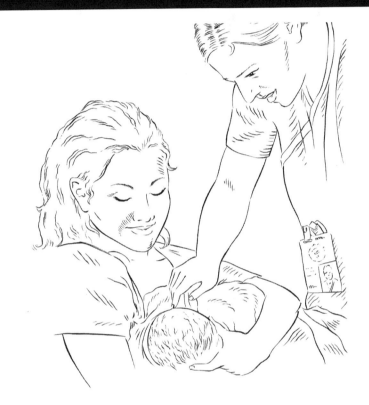

OBJECTIVES

By the end of this chapter, you will be able to:

• Understand and use vocabulary and phrases related to latch

• Give basic commands

• Count from 31 to 100

• Recognize colors

🎧 DIALOGUE

In this dialogue, a lactation consultant is helping a mother and her two-day-old baby get a comfortable and effective latch. They are in the mother's hospital room. Listen to the dialogue as you read along in the book. Repeat each line, pausing the audio as necessary; then listen to the vocabulary and important phrases, and repeat each one.

Setting:
• **Postpartum hospital room**

Characters:
• **Lactation consultant (Michelle)**
• **Mother (Ana)**
• **2-day-old baby**

LC: Buenos días! Me llamo Michelle. Soy consultora de lactancia. Tengo entendido que usted tiene dolor cuando amamanta.
[Good morning! My name is Michelle. I'm a lactation consultant. I understand that you're having pain with breastfeeding.]

Mother: Sí, me duele mucho cuando alimento a mi bebé. Tengo los pezones adoloridos.
[Yes, it hurts a lot when I feed my baby. I have sore nipples.]

LC: Lo siento mucho. ¿Desea ayudar a la bebé a pegarse al pecho ahora?

[I'm sorry to hear that. Do you want to help the baby latch onto the breast now?]

Mother: Sí, por favor.

[Yes, please.]

LC: ¿Está bien que le toque el pecho y a la bebé?

[Is it okay if I touch your breast and your baby?]

Mother: Sí, está bien.

[Yes, that's fine.]

LC: Muy bien. Vamos a comenzar con la bebé piel con piel en su pecho.

[Very good. Let's start with the baby skin-to-skin on your chest.]

Mother: Está buscando el pecho.

[She's looking for the breast.]

LC: ¡Excelente! Ahora vamos a ponerla panza con panza con su nariz contra el pezón.

[Great! Now let's help her get tummy-to-tummy and nose to nipple.]

Mother: OK.

[Okay.]

LC: Ahora vamos a ayudarla a pegarse al pecho con el pezón muy atrás en su boca. Eso hace que la lactancia sea más cómoda.

[Now let's help her get latched on so that your nipple is far back in her mouth. That makes breastfeeding more comfortable.]

Mother: Ya veo.

[I see.]

LC: Ahora deje que la cabeza de la bebé se incline hacia atrás y toque su labio inferior contra el pecho, pero lejos del pezón, un par de veces.

[Now let her head tilt back and touch her lower lip to the breast a few times, far from the nipple.]

Mother: Oh, ¡mire cómo abre la boca!

[Oh, look how she's opening her mouth!]

LC: Sí. Debe abrir la boca grande como un bostezo. Cuando ve eso, acérquela al pecho—no se acerque el pecho a la bebé.

[Yes. She should open her mouth wide like a yawn. When you see that, bring her to the breast—not the breast to the baby.]

Mother: OK. ¡Ahí está!

[Okay (baby latches on). There!]

LC: ¿Cómo se siente eso? ¿Le duele?

[How does that feel? Does it hurt?]

Mother: Bueno, lo puedo sentir, pero no me duele. No como antes.

[Well, I can feel it, but it doesn't hurt. Not like before.]

LC: Bien, ahora mire sus labios. ¿Puede ver que los labios se parecen a los de un pez? Si el labio inferior no se parece así, puede jalarle la barbilla para sacarlo.
[Good. Now look at her lips. Can you see that they look like the lips of a fish? If her lower lip doesn't look like that, you can tug her chin to pull it out.]

Mother: Sí, lo veo.
[Yes, I see that.]

LC: ¿Puede ver que la barbilla está muy hundida en su pecho y la nariz no toca el pecho?
[Can you see that her chin is very deep in your breast and her nose is off the breast?]

Mother: ¿Eso está bien?
[Is that good?]

LC: ¡Sí! Ahora, cuando termine de comer, introduzca el dedo en su boca para desprenderla. Puede poner un poco de leche en los pezones después de lactar para ayudar a la piel a curarse.
[Yes! Now when she's finished, stick your finger in her mouth to take her off the breast. You can put some milk on your nipples after the feeding to help the skin heal.]

IMPORTANT PHRASES

1. Tengo entendido que .... I understand that, I've been told that.

2. Un par de veces .... A couple of times.

3. ¿Cómo se siente eso? .... How does that feel?

4. ¿Dónde le duele? .... Where does it hurt?

5. ¿Le duele? .. .. Does it hurt?

6. Lo siento mucho .... I'm very sorry.

7. Lo puedo sentir .... I can feel it.

8. ¿Cómo deben estar? .... How should they be?

9. ¿Puede ver que…? .... Can you see that…?

10. ¡Ahí está! .. .. There!

11. Acerque al bebé al pecho,   Bring the baby to the breast,
    no el pecho al bebé .... not the breast to the baby.

VOCABULARY	
1. abrir	to open
2. acercar	to bring close
3. adolorido	sore, painful
4. alimentar	to feed
5. atrás	back
6. bostezo	yawn
7. como antes	like before
8. cómodo	comfortable
9. consejera de lactancia	lactation counselor
10. consultora de lactancia	lactation consultant
11. curarse	to heal
12. deber	should
13. dedo	finger
14. dejar	to let, to leave
15. desprender	to take off (the breast)
16. doler	to hurt
17. dolor	pain
18. enganche, agarre	latch
19. hundido	sunk into
20. inclinarse hacia atrás	to tilt, to lean back
21. introducir	to introduce, to put in
22. mirar	to look at
23. parecer	to look like, to seem, to appear
24. pez	fish
25. piel	skin
26. por favor	please
27. sentir, sentirse	to feel
28. terminar	to finish
29. tocar	to touch
30. tratar de	to try to

COMPREHENSION QUESTIONS

Exercise 1. After reading and listening to the dialogue on the audio file, listen again without the text and answer the following questions.

Note: If you are completing the exercises in this chapter for CERPs, write your answers on the answer sheets provided in Appendix A.

1. What problem does Ana say she is having?
Tengo...

   a. dolor de cabeza

   b. pezones adoloridos

   c. sueño

   d. dolor de espalda

2. Where should the nipple be located for a comfortable latch?
El pezón debe estar...

   a. en la mano

   b. en la boca

   c. muy atrás en la boca del bebé

   d. en el pecho

3. How should the baby's mouth be before latching on?
Debe abrir la boca grande como...

   a. un bostezo

   b. un pez

   c. un estómago

   d. una mano

4. How should the baby's lips look?
Los labios se parecen a los de...

   a. un bebé

   b. un pez

   c. una mamá

   d. la enfermera

5. What else can Ana do to alleviate sore nipples?
Puede poner un poco de _____ en los pezones después de lactar para ayudar la piel a curarse.

   a. pez

   b. comida

   c. leche

   d. pañal

LANGUAGE LESSONS

A. FORMAL COMMANDS

Just as there are two ways in Spanish to say "you" (the informal *tú* and the formal *usted*), there are both formal and informal commands, or ways to give instructions. In the medical setting, it is best to use a "formal" command. The formal command is easier to conjugate, with a small spelling change in the first person (*yo*) form of the verb in the present tense, which you studied in Chapter 2.

Singular formal commands (instructions directed at only one person) are created by conjugating the verb in the present tense *yo* form, then dropping the ending and adding an "*e*" to the stem of -*ar* verbs and an "*a*" to -*er* and -*ir* verbs. For example:

Tomar $\longrightarrow$ Tomo $\longrightarrow$ Tom $\longrightarrow$ Tome

1. *–ar* Verbs

- Tomar *[to take]*: Tome asiento, por favor. *[Please take a seat.]*
- Mirar *[to look]*: Mire la boca del bebé. *[Look at the baby's mouth.]*

2. *–er* and *–ir* Verbs

- Desprender *[to detach, take off]*: Desprenda al bebé del pecho.
  [Take the baby off the breast.]

- Abrir *[to open]*: Abra la boca. *[Open your mouth.]*

Exercise 2. Conjugate the verbs as singular formal commands in the following sentences.

1. Pase, Sra. González, y _____ (tomar) asiento.
   [Come in, Mrs. Gonzalez, and take a seat.]

2. _____ (mirar) la posición del bebé.
   [Look at the position of the baby.]

3. _____ (desprender) al bebé del pecho.
   [Take the baby off the breast.]

4. _____ (alimentar) a la bebé a demanda.
   [Feed the baby on cue.]

5. _____(tratar) de alimentar al bebé al menos ocho a 12 veces cada 24 horas.
   [Try to feed the baby at least eight to 12 times every 24 hours.]

3. SOME EXCEPTIONS

Some of the most common irregular commands and those with spelling changes are conjugated for you below with examples. A verb that has an irregular first-person conjugation will also be irregular as a formal command.

UNCONJUGATED	COMMAND	EXAMPLES
Ir *[to go]*	Vaya	Vaya al médico. *[Go to the doctor.]*
Hacer *[to do, to make]*	Haga	Haga una cita con la consultora de lactancia. *[Make an appointment with the lactation consultant.]*
Poner *[to put, to place]*	Ponga	Ponga al bebé nariz contra el pezón. *[Place the baby nose to nipple.]*
Comenzar *[to begin]*	Comience	Comience con el bebé "piel con piel." *[Start with the baby skin-to-skin.]*
Seguir *[to follow]*	Siga	Siga estos pasos para una buena posición y enganche. *[Follow these steps for a good position and latch.]*
Decir *[to say, to tell]*	Diga	Dígame cómo se siente. *[Tell me how you feel.]*
Sostener *[to hold]*	Sostenga	Sostenga al bebé muy cerca. *[Hold the baby very close.]*
Acercar *[to bring close]*	Acerque	Acerque al bebé al pecho. *[Bring the baby to the breast.]*

Exercise 3. Conjugate the irregular verbs as singular formal commands in the following sentences.

1. _____ (acercar) al bebé al pecho.
   [Bring the baby to the breast.]

2. _____ (hacer) una cita con el doctor.
   [Make an appointment with the doctor.]

3. _____ (ir) al hospital.
   [Go to the hospital.]

4. _____ (sostener) al bebé muy cerca.
   [Hold the baby very close.]

5. _____ (seguir) estos pasos para un buen enganche.
   [Follow these steps for a good latch.]

6. _____ (poner) al bebé panza con panza.
   [Place the baby tummy-to-tummy.]

7. _____ (comenzar) con una buena posición.
   [Start with a good position.]

B. Numbers 31-100

Listen to the speaker read the numbers from 31 to 40 and by tens up to 100, and repeat each one.

31: treinta y uno	35: treinta y cinco	39: treinta y nueve	70: setenta
32: treinta y dos	36: treinta y seis	40: cuarenta	80: ochenta
33: treinta y tres	37: treinta y siete	50: cincuenta	90: noventa
34: treinta y cuatro	38: treinta y ocho	60: sesenta	100: cien

Note that the numbers from forty to one hundred repeat the same pattern that we see in 31-39. You need only add *y uno, y dos,* etc.

Exercise 4. Listen as the speaker reads 10 numbers in Spanish; then write the numbers in the spaces below.

1._____ 3. _____ 5. _____ 7. _____ 9. _____

2. _____ 4. _____ 6. _____ 8. _____ 10. _____

 ## C. Colors

Listen to the speaker read the names of colors and repeat each one.

blanco: white	amarillo: yellow	morado: purple
rojo: red	verde: green	marrón: brown
anaranjado: orange	azul: blue	negro: black

Review: Days, Months, and Dates

 Exercise 5. Review the section in Chapter 2 on days of the week and months of the year. Practice writing and saying out loud the dates marked on the calendars below, including the day of the week.

JUNIO

D	L	M	M	J	V	S
			1	2	3	4
5 **1**	6	7	8	9	10 **4**	11
12	13	14	15	16	17	18
19	20	21	22	23	24	25
26	27	28	29	30	31	

JULIO

D	L	M	M	J	V	S
	1	2	3	4	5	6
7	8	9	10	11	12	13
14	15	16	17	18	19	20
21	22 **3**	23	24	25	26	27
28	29	30				

AGOSTO

D	L	M	M	J	V	S
				1	2	3
4 **2**	5	6	7	8	9	10
11	12	13	14	15	16	17
18	19	20	21	22	23	24
25	26	27	28	29	30	31 **5**

1. _____

2. _____

3. _____

4. _____

5. _____

🎧 LISTENING COMPREHENSION

Exercise 6. Listen to the dialogue on the audio file between a nurse and the mother of a newborn as they discuss latch; then answer the comprehension questions in English.

1. How did the mother place the baby to start the feeding?

_____

2. How was the baby's nose aligned?

_____

3. What did the baby do when his chin was touched to the breast?

_____

4. How did it feel to the mother when the baby latched on?

_____

Exercise 7. Breastfeeding Intake Exercise

In this exercise, you will listen to a conversation between a mother and a breastfeeding support person. The support person is gathering information about the mother and baby to complete an intake form. Listen to their conversation. Fill in the answers on the intake form in English.

Breastfeeding Intake Form

1. Mother's name _____

2. Baby's name _____

3. Phone number _____

4. Pediatrician _____

5. Baby's birthdate _____

TEAR-OUT QUICK REFERENCE: LATCH

KEY VOCABULARY	
ENGLISH	**SPANISH**
latch	enganche, agarre
to latch on	pegarse al pecho
to bring close	acercar
to take off (the breast)	desprender
pain	dolor

SINGULAR FORMAL COMMANDS		
ENGLISH	**SPANISH**	**EXAMPLE**
Go	Vaya	Vaya al hospital.
Take	Tome	Tome asiento, por favor.
Place, Put	Ponga	Ponga al bebé "panza con panza."
Say	Diga	Dígame cómo se siente.
Make	Haga	Haga una cita con el médico.
Hold	Sostenga	Sostenga al bebé muy cerca.
Begin	Comience	Comience con el bebé piel con piel.
Use	Use	Use una almohada.
Bring close	Acerque	Acerque al bebé al pecho.

COLORS	
ENGLISH	**SPANISH**
white	blanco
red	rojo
orange	anaranjado
yellow	amarillo
green	verde
blue	azul
purple	morado
brown	marrón
black	negro

COMMON PHRASES	
ENGLISH	**SPANISH**
How does that feel?	¿Cómo se siente eso?
Does it hurt?	¿Le duele?
Look at the baby's lips. They look like a fish's lips.	Mire los labios del bebé. Se parecen a los de un pez.
Can you see that…?	¿Puede ver que…?
You're doing very well!	¡Lo hace muy bien!
I understand that…	Tengo entendido que…
I'm very sorry.	Lo siento mucho.
Take him off the breast.	Despréndalo del pecho.
Bring the baby to the breast, not the breast to the baby.	Acerque al bebé al pecho, no el pecho al bebé.

Notes for the Classroom Instructor

This section is for instructors using this book in a classroom setting.

Section A: Formal Commands

The teaching of commands provides many opportunities for classroom activities in groups and in pairs. Some suggestions include:

1. After presenting some basic commands, play "Simon Says" with the class as a whole, using "*Toquen el/la...*" "*Levanten el/la...*", etc. This is a great way to practice plural commands and review recently learned anatomy terms.

2. The "Simon Says" exercise can be turned around, with students issuing commands to the teacher to practice singular commands. This can be done in Round Robin style, with each student taking a turn. Of course, the teacher only obeys correctly conjugated commands, but students can help and correct each other.

3. Students can work in pairs and practice giving each other commands for achieving a good latch. They can write the dialogue down, and then practice with each other, or you can ask them to improvise, using the various dialogues from the chapter as a guide.

ANSWER KEY

Need help with these exercises? Looking for more opportunities to practice? For support and additional resources to help you learn to provide breastfeeding support in Spanish, visit www.spanishforbreastfeedingsupport.com.

Exercise 1.

1. b

2. c

3. a

4. b

5. c

Exercise 2.

1. tome

2. Mire

3. Desprenda

4. Alimente

5. Trate

Exercise 3.

1. Acerque

2. Haga

3. Vaya

4. Sostenga

5. Siga

6. Ponga

7. Comience

Exercise 4.

1. 38

2. 99

3. 45

4. 62

5. 71

6. 56

7. 83

8. 37

9. 100

10. 34

Exercise 5.

1. domingo, el cinco de junio

2. domingo, el cuatro de agosto

3. lunes, el veintidós de julio

4. viernes, el diez de junio

5. sábado, el treinta y uno de agosto

Listening Comprehension Dialogue

Nurse: Comencemos con el bebé piel con piel contra su pecho.
[Let's start with the baby skin-to-skin on your chest.]

Mother: O, está buscando el pecho.
[Oh, he's looking for the breast.]

Nurse: Bien. Ponga al bebé nariz contra el pezón.
[Good. Line him up nose to nipple.]

Mother: ¿Así?
[Like this?]

Nurse: Sí. Ahora toque su barbilla contra el pecho.
[Yes. Now touch his chin to the breast.]

Mother: Está abriendo la boca grande.
[He's opening wide.]

Nurse: Muy bien. Cuando tiene la boca muy abierta, acérquelo al pecho.
[Great. When his mouth is open wide, bring him to the breast.]

Mother: ¡O, sí, ahí está!
[Oh, yes, there!]

Nurse: ¿Le duele?
[Does that hurt?]

Mother: No. Lo puedo sentir, pero no me duele.
[No. I can feel it, but it doesn't hurt.]

Exercise 6.

1. Skin-to-skin, against her chest

2. Nose to nipple

3. He is opening his mouth wide.

4. She could feel it, but it didn't hurt.

Intake Dialogue

Q: Hola. ¿Cómo se llama?

A: Me llamo Yessica Díaz.

Q: ¿Cómo se llama su bebé?

A: Se llama Selena Martínez.

Q: ¿Cuál es su número de teléfono?

A: Es el (232) 875-0234.

Q: ¿Cómo se llama el doctor de su bebé?

A: Se llama el Dr. López.

Q: ¿Cuándo nació la bebé?

A: El ocho de octubre.

Exercise 7.

1. Mother's name: Yessica (or Jessica) Díaz

2. Baby's name: Selena Martínez

3. Phone number: (232) 875-0234

4. Pediatrician: Dr. Lopez

5. Baby's birthdate: October 8

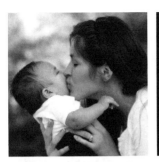

CHAPTER 4
FEEDING FREQUENCY AND DURATION

OBJECTIVES

By the end of this chapter, you will be able to:

• Understand and use vocabulary and phrases related to feeding frequency and duration

• Describe people and things

• Use *ser* and *estar* and understand the difference

• Use question words

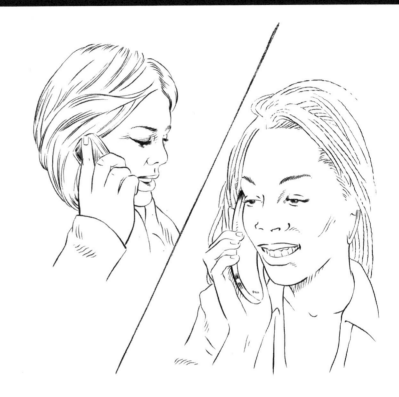

🎧 DIALOGUE

In this dialogue, a breastfeeding peer counselor answers a breastfeeding support hotline and talks with the mother of a 10-day-old baby about feeding frequency and duration. Listen to the dialogue as you read along in the book. Repeat each line, pausing the audio as necessary; then listen to the vocabulary and important phrases, and repeat each one.

Setting:
• **WIC office and mother calling in from home**

Characters:
• **WIC Breastfeeding Peer Counselor (Roxanne)**
• **Mother (Marisol)**
• **10-day-old baby**

PC: Hola, línea de apoyo a la lactancia. ¿Cómo puedo ayudarla?
[Hello, breastfeeding support line. How can I help you?]

Mother: Hola, me llamo Marisol. Estoy llamando porque mi bebé come con mucha frecuencia y estoy preocupada.
[Hello, this is Marisol. I'm calling because my baby is eating very often, and I'm worried.]

NOTES

PC: Hola Marisol. Me llamo Roxanne. ¿Puedo hacerle unas preguntas acerca de usted y su bebé? (fills out form with information) Y, ¿cómo está creciendo la bebé?
[Hi Marisol, this is Roxanne. Can I ask some questions about you and your baby? (fills out form with information) And how is your baby growing?]

Mother: O, ¡ya está grande! El doctor dice que está creciendo muy bien. Aumentó nueve onzas la semana pasada. Ahora pesa siete libras con 10 onzas.
[Oh, she's big already! The doctor says she's growing very well. She gained nine ounces last week. Now she weighs seven pounds, 10 ounces.]

PC: ¡Muy bien! Y, ¿con qué frecuencia come la bebé?
[Great! And how often is your baby eating?]

Mother: Más o menos cada dos horas. A veces cada tres horas.
[About every two hours. Sometimes every three hours.]

PC: Bueno, es normal que los bebés coman con esa frecuencia. Necesitan comer al menos ocho a 12 veces cada 24 horas.
[Well, it's normal for babies to eat that often. They need to eat at least eight to 12 times in 24 hours.]

Mother: ¿Necesito darle un biberón con fórmula? Mi amiga dice que es mejor las dos cosas.
[Do I need to give her a bottle of formula? My friend said it's best to give her both breastmilk and formula.]

PC: No es necesario usar fórmula. Ella está creciendo muy bien con su leche, y mi doctor dice que es más saludable para ella recibir sólo la leche materna. El usar fórmula también puede reducir la cantidad de leche que su cuerpo produce.
[There's no need to use formula. She's growing very well on your milk, and my doctor says it's healthier for her to have only breastmilk. Using formula can also reduce your milk supply.]

Mother: Trato de alimentarla a demanda. Pero a veces dura mucho tiempo comiendo.
[I'm trying to feed her on cue. But sometimes she takes a long time to eat.]

PC: Entiendo. Sugiero que observe a su bebé y no el reloj. Cuando está comiendo, traga la leche. Cuando sólo busca consuelo, succiona, pero no traga mucho.
[I understand. I suggest watching your baby, not the clock. When your baby is eating, you see lots of swallows. When she's nursing for comfort you see lots of sucking, but not many swallows.]

Mother: ¿Cómo puedo saber la diferencia?
[How can I tell the difference?]

PC: Cuando la bebé traga, hace un movimiento lento con la mandíbula. A veces se escucha un sonido también, como un "kh."
[When your baby is swallowing, she moves her jaw slowly. Sometimes you can hear a little sound, too, like this, "kh."]

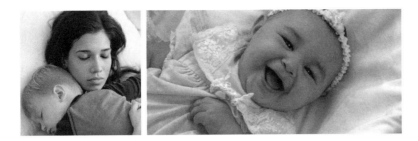

Mother: ¿Siempre debo ofrecerle los dos pechos?
[Should I always offer both breasts?]

PC: Es una buena idea ofrecerle los dos pechos, especialmente con una bebé recién nacida. Está bien si no toma del segundo pecho.
[It's a good idea to offer both, especially with a newborn. It's okay if she doesn't take the second breast.]

Mother: ¿Cómo puedo saber cuando termina de comer?
[How do I know when she's done?]

PC: Puede desprenderse sola, o dormirse. Si busca consuelo después de recibir suficiente leche, está bien quitarla del pecho.
[Your baby might come off on her own, or fall asleep. If she's nursing for comfort after getting plenty of milk, it's okay to take her off.]

Mother: Muchas gracias por su ayuda.
[Thank you very much for your help.]

IMPORTANT PHRASES

1. Trato de .... I try to.

2. ¿Con qué frecuencia? .... How often?

3. Las dos cosas* .... both things (breastfeeding and formula feeding)

4. Alimentar a demanda .... to feed on cue, on demand

5. Más o menos .... more or less, about

6. Eso es normal .... That's normal.

7. Al menos ocho a   At least eight to
   12 veces cada 24 horas .... 12 times in 24 hours.

8. Cada 2 a 3 horas .... Every 2 to 3 hours.

9. Sugiero que observe   I suggest you watch
   a su bebé y no el reloj .... the baby, not the clock.

10. Muchas gracias por su ayuda ...... Thank you very much for your help.

* This is a colloquial expression that may or may not be used in your community.

VOCABULARY

1. a veces .... sometimes
2. al nacer .... at birth
3. amigo/a .... friend
4. aumentar .... to gain weight
5. biberón .... bottle
6. cada .... each, every
7. comer .... to eat
8. consuelo .... comfort
9. crecer .... to grow
10. dar, darle .... to give
11. diferencia .... difference
12. dormirse .... to fall asleep
13. durar .... to last, to take a long time
14. escuchar .... to hear
15. fórmula .... formula
16. frecuencia .... frequency
17. grande .... big
18. horas .... hours
19. lento .... slow
20. libra .. .. pound
21. mejor .... better, best
22. movimiento .... movement
23. mucho .... a lot
24. necesitar .... to need
25. necesario .... necessary
26. normal .... normal
27. ofrecer .... to offer
28. onza .... ounce
29. pesar .... to weigh
30. preocupado/a .... worried
31. quitar .... to take off
32. recién nacido/a .... newborn
33. reducir .... to reduce, to lower
34. reloj .... clock, watch
35. saber .... to know (a fact)
36. saludable .... healthy
37. segundo .... second
38. sonido .... sound
39. succionar .... to suck
40. sugerir .... to suggest
41. también .... also
42. tanto .... so much
43. tomar .... to take, to drink
44. tragar .... to swallow

COMPREHENSION QUESTIONS

Exercise 1. After reading and listening to the dialogue on the audio file, listen again without the text and answer the following questions in Spanish. Don't worry about forming complete sentences; simply focus on writing down the key information.

Note: If you are completing the exercises in this chapter for CERPs, write your answers on the answer sheets provided in Appendix A.

1. What is Marisol's concern?

   _____

2. How does the doctor say that the baby is growing?

   _____

3. How often is Marisol's baby eating?

   _____

4. How can Marisol tell whether her baby is eating or nursing for comfort?

   _____

5. How can Marisol tell that her baby is done with a feeding?

   _____

LANGUAGE LESSONS

A. DESCRIBING PEOPLE AND THINGS

In Spanish, the describing word (adjective) generally follows the object or person it describes. So, instead of "a happy baby," in Spanish we would say the equivalent of "a baby happy."

Adjectives reflect the gender and number of the person or object in their spelling. Here are some examples:

Masculine Nouns and Adjectives

- El bebé pesad**o** *[the heavy baby]*
- Los movimientos lent**os** *[the slow movements]*

Feminine Nouns and Adjectives

- La bebé desnud**a** *[the naked baby]*
- La mamá cansad**a** *[the tired mother]*
- Las tomas larg**as** *[the long feedings]*

Note: Adjectives ending in "*e*" or a consonant do not change according to gender. Examples: *grande* (big), *feliz* (happy), *interesante* (interesting), *importante* (important)

- El hospital grande *[the big hospital]*
- El bebé feliz (or la bebé feliz) *[the happy baby]*
- Las instrucciones importantes *[the important instructions]*

Exercise 2. Match the following nouns with the appropriate adjective.

1. el hospital	a. lento
2. la bebé	b. largas
3. las madres	c. cansadas
4. el movimiento	d. adoloridos
5. los pezones	e. grande
6. las tomas	f. pesada

B. To Be: *Ser* and *Estar*

Both *ser* and *estar* translate as "to be" in Spanish. The Spanish language divides the concept of "to be" into two categories: *ser* is used to describe identity, permanent conditions, or what something is, while *estar* is generally used with temporary emotions and conditions, location, or how something is. Let's begin with the present tense conjugation of *ser* and *estar*, which are both irregular:

SER		ESTAR	
Yo: **Soy**	Nosotros: **Somos**	Yo: **Estoy**	Nosotros: **Estamos**
Tú: **Eres**		Tú: **Estás**	
Él, Ella, Usted: **Es**	Ellos, Ustedes: **Son**	Él, Ella, Usted: **Está**	Ellos, Ustedes: **Están**

Examples:

- Soy enfermera. *[I am a nurse.]*
- Estoy cansada. *[I am tired.]*

You can see from the above examples that *ser* is used to describe one's profession, while *estar* is used to describe temporary conditions like being tired. The following table indicates the most common uses for *ser* and *estar* in the breastfeeding context, with examples for each.

SER		ESTAR	
Profession	Ellas son enfermeras *[They are nurses.]*	**Location**	Estamos en el hospital. *[We are in the hospital.]* El bebé está en la posición de cuna. *[The baby is in the cradle hold.]*
Relationship	Ella es mi madre. *[She is my mother.]*	**Emotion**	Estoy feliz. *[I am happy.]*
National Origin/ Nationality	Sara es de Francia. *[Sara is from France.]* Sara es francesa. *[Sara is French.]*	**Condition**	Las madres están cansadas. *[The mothers are tired.]*

Exercise 3. Conjugate *ser* or *estar* in the following sentences.

1. Elena no _____ (estar) en el hospital.
   [*Elena is not in the hospital.*]

2. Nosotras _____ (estar) felices de amamantar a nuestros bebés.
   [*We are happy to be breastfeeding our babies.*]

3. Usted _____ (ser) una doctora excelente.
   [*You are an excellent doctor.*]

4. Mi hermana y yo _____ (ser) mexicanas.
   [*My sister and I are Mexican.*]

5. Yo _____ (ser) la mamá del bebé.
   [*I am the baby's mother.*]

Exercise 4. Fill in the blanks with the proper form of either *ser* or *estar*.

1. A veces las mamás _____ cansadas.
   [*Sometimes, mothers are tired.*]

2. Yo _____ consejera de lactancia.
   [*I am a lactation counselor.*]

3. Marta _____ de Argentina.
   [*Marta is from Argentina.*]

4. La bebé _____ feliz hoy.
   [*The baby is happy today.*]

5. Nosotros _____ colombianos.
   [*We are Colombian.*]

C. QUESTION WORDS

The following words are used to ask questions:

¿Quién?/¿Quiénes?	Who?	**¿Por qué?**	Why?
¿Qué?/¿Cuál?/¿Cuáles?	What?/Which?	**¿Cómo?**	How?
¿Cuándo?	When?	**¿Dónde?**	Where?
¿Cuánto?/¿Cuántos? ¿Cuánta?/¿Cuántas?	How many?	**¿Cuánto/¿Cuánta?**	How much?

Note: All question words require an accent mark.

Examples:

- **¿Cómo** puedo ayudarla hoy? *[How can I help you today?]*
- **¿Qué** parte del bebé toca el pecho primero? *[What part of the baby touches the breast first?]*
- **¿Dónde** está la oficina de la consultora de lactancia? *[Where is the lactation consultant's office?]*

Note: When using *cuánto* before a noun, it must agree with the noun in gender and number. For example:

- ¿Cuán**ta** leche necesita el bebé? *[How much milk does the baby need?]*
- ¿Cuán**tos** doctores están en el hospital? *[How many doctors are in the hospital?]*

By contrast, when *cuánto* is used before a verb, it remains singular and masculine. For example:

- **¿Cuánto** come la bebé? *[How much does the baby eat?]*
- **¿Cuánto** pesa el bebé? *[How much does the baby weigh?]*

Other question words agree in number only. For example:

- ¿Quién es su doctor? *[Who is your doctor?]*
- ¿Quién**es** son los padres? *[Who are the parents?]*
- ¿Cuál es su fecha de nacimiento? *[What is your birth date?]*
- ¿Cuál**es** son sus sugerencias acerca del uso del chupón? *[What are your suggestions about the use of a pacifier?]*

Exercise 5. Fill in the blanks with the appropriate question word.

1. ¿ _____ se siente hoy?

2. ¿ _____ significa "piel con piel"?

3. ¿ _____ es su fecha de nacimiento?

4. ¿ _____ leche necesita el bebé?

5. ¿ _____ pesa la bebé?

LANGUAGE REVIEW: COMMANDS

Exercise 6. Use the list of verbs below to write a short series of commands to guide a mother in achieving proper latch and positioning. Review the vocabulary and commands from Chapter 3.

1. Sostener _____

2. Dejar _____

3. Mirar _____

4. Acercar _____

_____

_____

🎧 LISTENING COMPREHENSION

Exercise 7. Listen to the dialogue on the audio file between a mother and a lactation consultant as they discuss feeding frequency and weight gain; then answer the comprehension questions in English.

1. Why has the mother come to see the lactation consultant?

   _____

2. How often is the baby eating?

   _____

3. What does the lactation consultant tell her about feeding frequency?

   _____

4. How is the mother deciding when to feed the baby?

   _____

5. What did the doctor say about the baby?

   _____

Exercise 8. Breastfeeding Intake Exercise

In this exercise, you will listen to a conversation between a mother and a breastfeeding support person. The support person is gathering information about the mother and baby to complete an intake form. Listen to their conversation. Fill in the answers on the intake form in English.

Breastfeeding Intake Form

1. Mother's name   _____

2. Baby's name   _____

3. Phone number   _____

4. Pediatrician   _____

5. Baby's birthdate   _____

6. Baby's birth weight   _____

7. Number of feedings in 24 hours _____

8. Formula use (yes/no) _____

9. Amount   _____

TEAR-OUT QUICK REFERENCE: FEEDING FREQUENCY AND DURATION

COMMON ADJECTIVES

ENGLISH	SPANISH
slow	lento
tired	cansado
big	grande
small	pequeño
perfect	perfecto
special	especial

SER / ESTAR

SER		ESTAR	
Profession	Ellas son enfermeras *[They are nurses.]*	**Location**	Estamos en el hospital. *[We are in the hospital.]* El bebé está en la posición de cuna. *[The baby is in the cradle hold.]*
Relationship	Ella es mi madre. *[She is my mother.]*	**Emotion**	Estoy feliz. *[I am happy.]*
National Origin/ Nationality	Sara es de Francia. *[Sara is from France.]* Sara es francesa. *[Sara is French.]*	**Condition**	Las madres están cansadas. *[The mothers are tired.]*

QUESTION WORDS

¿Quién?/¿Quiénes?	Who?	**¿Por qué?**	Why?
¿Qué?/¿Cuál?/¿Cuáles?	What?/Which?	**¿Cómo?**	How?
¿Cuándo?	When?	**¿Dónde?**	Where?
¿Cuánto?/¿Cuántos? ¿Cuánta?/¿Cuántas?	How many?	**¿Cuánto/¿Cuánta?**	How much?

COMMON PHRASES

ENGLISH	SPANISH
How often does the baby eat?	¿Con qué frecuencia come el bebé?
That is normal.	Eso es normal.
Babies need to eat at least eight to 12 times every 24 hours.	Los bebés necesitan comer al menos ocho a 12 veces cada 24 horas.
When the baby is eating, she swallows the milk.	Cuando la bebé come, traga la leche.
When he only wants comfort, he will suck but not swallow very much.	Cuando sólo busca consuelo succiona, pero no traga mucho.
When the baby swallows, he makes a slow movement with his jaw.	Cuando el bebé traga, hace un movimiento lento de la mandíbula.
Sometimes, you can also hear a sound.	A veces se escucha un sonido también.
Try to feed the baby on cue.	Trate de alimentar al bebé a demanda.

NOTES FOR THE CLASSROOM INSTRUCTOR

This section is for instructors using this book in a classroom setting.

SECTIONS A AND B: ADJECTIVES, *SER/ESTAR*

1. A fun classroom activity is to have each student write three adjectives that describe him/her on a piece of paper, collect all the descriptions and read them to the class, allowing the students to guess who is being described. This exercise also can be modified to describe objects in the classroom.

2. To combine adjective practice with *ser* and *estar*, ask the students to write 3-5 descriptive sentences about themselves, collect the descriptions, and read them to the class. Have the students guess whom the sentences are describing.

3. Another activity that combines adjectives with *ser* and *estar* is 20 Questions. There are many variations on 20 Questions that can be played in the classroom, either in pairs, small groups, or as a whole class with the teacher. Students can guess objects in the room, other students, or objects used on the job.

4. Another participatory activity is to have the students bring to class an object they use in their work (breast pump, scale, dropper, nipple shields) and describe it for the class using *ser*. A variation on this activity would be to have the students hide their objects while describing them and make the class guess. Or, they can simply think of an object they use at work and describe it for the other students.

SECTION C: QUESTION WORDS

Surveys are a good way to get students involved in using question words. You can create a short survey using as many question words as possible. Have the students work in pairs, asking each other the questions and writing the answers down. Then you can ask each student to introduce their partner to the class, providing information gained from the survey.

Answer Key

Need help with these exercises? Looking for more opportunities to practice? For support and additional resources to help you learn to provide breastfeeding support in Spanish, visit www.spanishforbreastfeedingsupport.com.

Exercise 1.

1. la bebé come con mucha frecuencia

2. está creciendo muy bien

3. cada dos horas, más o menos, a veces cada tres horas

4. cuando come, traga la leche, hace un movimiento lento con la mandíbula, se escucha un sonido

5. desprenderse sola, o dormirse

Exercise 2.

1. e
2. f
3. c
4. a
5. d
6. b

Exercise 3.

1. está
2. estamos
3. es
4. somos
5. soy

Exercise 4.

1. están
2. soy
3. es
4. está
5. somos

Exercise 5.

1. Cómo
2. Qué
3. Cuál
4. Cuánta
5. Cuánto

Exercise 6.

Answers will vary, but some possible commands include:

1. Sostenga al bebé panza con panza (or piel con piel, or muy cerca de usted).

2. Deje que la cabeza de la bebé se incline hacia atrás.

3. Mire los labios del bebé.

4. Acerque al bebé al pecho.

Listening Comprehension Dialogue

Mother: Mi bebé come tanto.
[My baby eats so much.]

LC: ¿Con qué frecuencia?
[How often?]

Mother: Cada dos a tres horas.
[Every two to three hours.]

LC: Eso es normal. Los bebés necesitan comer al menos ocho a 12 veces en 24 horas.
[That sounds normal. Babies need to eat at least eight to 12 times every 24 hours.]

Mother: OK. Trato de alimentar a la bebé a demanda.
[Okay. I'm trying to feed the baby on cue.]

LC: ¿Está aumentando de peso su bebé?
[Is your baby gaining weight?]

Mother: O, sí. Dice el doctor que la bebé está bien.
[Oh, yes. The doctor says that the baby is fine.]

Exercise 7.

1. The baby is eating a lot.

2. Every two to three hours

3. This is normal; babies need to eat 8-12 times in 24 hours.

4. On cue/on demand

5. The baby is fine.

Intake Dialogue

Q: Hola. ¿Cómo se llama?
A: Me llamo Elena de Castillo.

Q: ¿Cómo se llama su bebé?
A: Se llama Rafael Castillo.

Q: ¿Cuál es su número de teléfono?
A: Es el (916) 758-4408.

Q: ¿Cómo se llama el doctor de su bebé?
A: Se llama la doctora Pérez.

Q: ¿Cuándo nació el bebé?
A: El nueve de marzo.

Q: ¿Cuánto pesó el bebé al nacer?
A: Pesó siete libras con tres onzas.

Q: ¿Cuántas veces alimenta al bebé en 24 horas?
A: 9 veces.

Q: ¿El bebé toma fórmula?
A: Sí, a veces.

Q: ¿Cuánta fórmula?
A: Un biberón con dos onzas por día.

Exercise 8.

1. Mother's name: Elena de Castillo

2. Baby's name: Rafael Castillo

3. Phone number: (916) 758-4408

4. Pediatrician: Doctora Pérez

5. Baby's birthdate: March 9

6. Baby's birth weight: 7 lbs., 3 ozs.

7. Number of feedings in 24 hours: 9 times

8. Formula use (yes/no): Yes

9. Amount: One bottle with two ounces per day

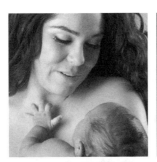

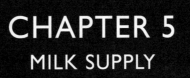

CHAPTER 5
MILK SUPPLY

OBJECTIVES

By the end of
this chapter, you
will be able to:

• Understand and
use vocabulary and
phrases related
to milk supply

• Describe things
happening in the
immediate present

• Use *saber* and *conocer*
and understand
the difference

• Make polite
recommendations
and suggestions

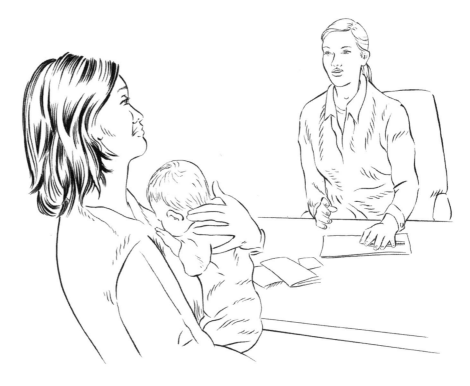

DIALOGUE

In this dialogue, a lactation consultant is discussing milk supply with the mother of a three-week-old baby at a breastfeeding clinic. Listen to the dialogue as you read along in the book. Repeat each line, pausing the audio as necessary; then listen to the vocabulary and important phrases, and repeat each one.

Setting:
• **Breastfeeding clinic**

Characters:
• **Lactation consultant (Laura)**

• **Mother (Cecilia)**

• **Three-week-old baby**

     LC: Hola Cecilia, ¿cómo está?
       [Hi Cecilia. How are you?]

Mother: No muy bien. El pediatra dice que mi bebé no está creciendo bien.
     [Not so well. The pediatrician says that my baby isn't growing well.]

LC: Lo siento mucho. ¿Cómo se siente usted?
[I'm sorry to hear that. How are you feeling?]

Mother: Me siento frustrada y preocupada.
[I feel frustrated and worried.]

LC: Usted se siente frustrada y preocupada—la entiendo. Otras madres tienen los mismos sentimientos.
[You feel frustrated and worried—I understand. Other mothers have the same feelings.]

Mother: ¿Hay algo que puedo hacer para incrementar la cantidad de leche que mi cuerpo produce?
[Is there anything I can do to increase my milk supply?]

LC: Sí hay. Cuando se despierte el bebé, veremos si se está prendiendo bien al pecho. ¿Con qué frecuencia está alimentando al bebé?
[Yes, there is. When the baby wakes up, we'll see if he's latching well. How often are you feeding him?]

Mother: Le estoy dando pecho más o menos cada tres horas. A veces cada cuatro horas de noche.
[I'm feeding him about every three hours. Sometimes every four hours at night.]

LC: La cantidad de leche que usted produce depende de un sistema de oferta y demanda. Trate de alimentar al bebé con más frecuencia— necesitan comer al menos ocho a 12 veces cada 24 horas.
[Milk supply is a supply and demand system. Try to feed him more often – they need to eat at least eight to 12 times every 24 hours.]

Mother: OK. Puedo hacer eso. Mi amiga dice que debo amamantarlo por diez minutos de cada lado. ¿Eso es correcto?
[Okay. I can do that. My friend says I should nurse him for ten minutes on each side. Is that right?]

LC: Bueno, al comienzo de la toma, su bebé recibe la leche inicial, una leche aguada que satisface la sed del bebé. Más tarde, recibe la leche final, que es rica en calorías y le ayuda a crecer. Por eso, recomiendo dejar al bebé en el primer pecho hasta que se duerma o él sólo se retire. Entonces, puede sacarle los gases al bebé y cambiarle al otro lado.
[Well, at the beginning of the feeding your baby gets the foremilk, which is watery and satisfies your baby's thirst. Later, he gets the hindmilk, which is rich in calories, to help him grow.So I recommend leaving the baby on the first breast until he falls asleep or comes off the breast. Then you can burp him and switch him to the other side.]

Mother: OK.
[Okay.]

LC: También puede apretar el pecho durante la alimentación, para sacarse más leche y aumentar la cantidad de leche.
[You can also squeeze your breast during the feeding, to get more milk out and to help your supply.]

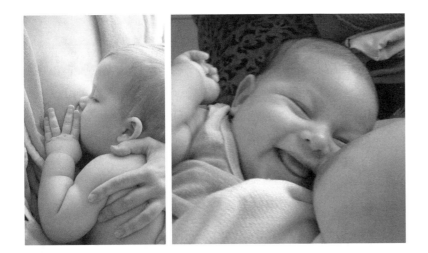

Mother: Perfecto. Puedo hacer eso también.
[Great. I can do that, too.]

LC: El extraer la leche después de amamantar también aumenta la cantidad de leche. Recomiendo usar un sacaleches calidad de hospital. Puede alquilar uno aquí.
[Pumping after feedings increases milk supply, too. I recommend using a hospital grade pump. You can rent one here.]

Mother: ¿Conoce algún alimento o hierba que pueda incrementar mi producción de leche?
[Do you know of any food or herb that can increase my supply?]

LC: Sí. Este papel indica cuáles alimentos y hierbas incrementan la producción de leche.
[Yes. This handout indicates which foods and herbs increase milk supply.]

Mother: Gracias. O, también estamos usando un chupón. ¿Está bien?
[Thank you. Oh, we're also using a pacifier. Is that okay?]

LC: Creo que debería dejar de usarlo por un rato.
[I think you should stop using it for awhile.]

IMPORTANT PHRASES

1. Vamos a ver .... Let's see.

2. Creo que debería .... I think you should.

3. Dejar de usarlo .... to stop using it

4. Lo siento mucho... I'm sorry to hear that.

5. ¿Cómo se siente usted? ....How do you feel?

6. Por un rato...for awhile

VOCABULARY

1. acerca de .... about
2. alquilar ....to rent
3. apretar ....to squeeze
4. calidad .... quality
5. cantidad de leche.......... amount of milk, milk supply
6. chupón.................................... pacifier
7. conocer ...... to know, to be familiar with
8. creer..to believe
9. decir (dice) .... to say
10. depender de .... to depend on
11. entonces ....so, then
12. frustrado/a........................... frustrated
13. grasa ....fat
14. hacer ....to make, to do
15. hierba...herb
16. incrementar .... to increase
17. leche final .... hindmilk
18. leche inicial .... foremilk
19. mayoría .... most
20. mismo/a..................................... same
21. oferta y demanda ... supply and demand
22. papel............................ paper, handout
23. pediatra ....pediatrician
24. prenderse ....to latch, to latch on
25. preocupado/a ....worried
26. producción de leche... milk production, milk supply
27. producir .... to produce
28. recomendar....................to recommend
29. rico...rich
30. saber .... to know (a fact)
31. sacaleches, tiraleches, bomba .... breastpump
32. sacarle los gases ....to burp (the baby)
33. sacarse ....to take out, to pump milk
34. sentimiento............................... feeling
35. si .... if, whether*
36. sistema...................................... system
37. tener.....................................to have

The word sí with an accent on the í means "yes," while si without an accent means "if" or "whether."

COMPREHENSION QUESTIONS

Exercise 1. After reading and listening to the dialogue on the audio file, listen again without the text and answer the following questions in Spanish. Don't worry about forming complete sentences; simply focus on writing down the key information.

Note: If you are completing the exercises in this chapter for CERPs, write your answers on the answer sheets provided in Appendix A.

1. What did Cecilia's doctor say about her baby?

   _____

2. How can Cecilia tell whether her baby is getting enough milk?

   _____

3. How often does she feed her baby?

   _____

4. What does the lactation consultant say that milk supply depends on?

   _____

5. What are two ways the lactation consultant suggests to increase milk production?

   _____

LANGUAGE LESSONS

A. WHAT'S HAPPENING RIGHT NOW (IMMEDIATE PRESENT TENSE)

The present tense, which you learned in Chapter 2, describes activities going on in the present moment or typical and recurring activities. Another way to express something that is happening at the time of speaking is with the present progressive tense. In English, the present progressive tense requires a word ending in –ing. For example:

PRESENT TENSE	PRESENT PROGRESSIVE
She eats	She is eating
Ella come	Ella está comiendo

In order to form the present progressive, we conjugate two different verbs. First, the verb *estar* (to be) is conjugated according to the person doing the action.

ESTAR	
Yo: **Estoy**	Nosotros: **Estamos**
Tú: **Estás**	
Él, Ella, Usted: **Está**	Ellos, Ustedes: **Están**

Examples:

• Ella **está** alimentando al bebé cada dos horas. *[She is feeding the baby every two hours.]*

• Las enfermeras **están** ayudando a la mamá. *[The nurses are helping the mother.]*

Second, we join the conjugated *estar* with another verb, which will have one of the following endings:

-AR VERBS	-ER/-IR VERBS
-ando	**-iendo**
Examples: ayudar - ayudando succionar - succionando buscar - buscando	Examples: comer - comiendo recibir - recibiendo abrir - abriendo

Examples:

• El bebé **está buscando** el pecho. *[The baby is looking for the breast.]*

• El bebé **está abriendo** la boca grande. *[The baby is opening his mouth wide.]*

Exercise 2. Conjugate the verbs in the immediate present in the following paragraph.

    Example: El bebé _____ (buscar) el pecho.

        El bebé **está buscando** el pecho.

Claudia está en la clínica de lactancia hoy. Ella _____ (amamantar) a su bebé de tres días, Ricardo. Claudia _____ (sostener) al bebé piel con piel. Las consultoras de lactancia _____ (ayudar) a Claudia a tener una buena posición. El bebé _____ (comer) suficiente leche y Claudia _____ (escuchar) un sonido cuando Ricardo come.

Note: Some verbs undergo a stem change or a spelling change when forming the immediate present. Two of the most common verbs with these changes are *decir—diciendo* and *ir—yendo*.

B. To Know: *Saber* and *Conocer*

In Spanish, there are two verbs to express "to know." The verb *saber* refers to knowing a fact, while *conocer* refers to being familiar with a person, place, or concept.

Both *saber* and *conocer* are irregular in the present tense first person (*yo*) form. The remaining conjugations are regular in the present tense.

SABER		CONOCER	
Yo: **Sé**	Nosotros: **Sabemos**	Yo: **Conozco**	Nosotros: **Conocemos**
Tú: **Sabes**		Tú: **Conoces**	
Él, Ella, Usted: **Sabe**	Ellos, Ustedes: **Saben**	Él, Ella, Usted: **Conocen**	Ellos, Ustedes: **Conocen**

Examples:

• **Sabemos** que es importante evitar la formula. *[We know that it is important to avoid formula.]*

• No **sé** si estoy produciendo suficiente leche. *[I don't know whether I am producing enough milk.]*

• **Conozco** a la consultora de lactancia de este hospital. *[I know the lactation consultant at this hospital.]*

Exercise 3. Conjugate *saber* or *conocer* in the present tense in the following sentences.

1. Las mamás _____ (saber) que los bebés necesitan comer al menos ocho a 12 veces en 24 horas.

2. Yo no _____ (conocer) a la consejera de lactancia.

3. Nosotros _____ (conocer) muchas técnicas para producir suficiente leche.

4. Ella no _____ (saber) lo que significa "piel con piel."

5. ¿_____ (conocer) usted la técnica de dar pecho a demanda?

Exercise 4. Fill in the blanks with the proper form in the present tense of either *saber* or *conocer*.

1. Nosotros _____ a una consejera de lactancia que puede ayudarla.

2. La consejera de lactancia _____ cómo ayudar a las mamás con los pezones adoloridos.

3. Las enfermeras _____ las técnicas para una buena producción de leche.

4. Yo no _____ lo que significa "alimentar a demanda."

5. Ella no _____ a la doctora.

C. Giving Instructions

In addition to formal commands, which you learned in Chapter 3, there are various phrases that will help you give polite instructions to breastfeeding mothers. This exercise summarizes some of the most common ways to make suggestions and recommendations.

- **Trate de**...*Try to...*

- **Recomiendo**...*I recommend...*

- **Usted puede**...*You can...*

- **Creo que debería**...*I think you should...*

Exercise 5. Match the statements above with the following endings in order to create a series of instructions and recommendations regarding milk supply.

1. _____ tener un buen enganche para incrementar la producción de leche.

2. _____ alimentar al bebé con más frecuencia.

3. _____ dejar al bebé en el primer pecho hasta que se duerma o él sólo se retire.

4. _____ apretar el pecho durante la alimentación.

5. _____ extraer la leche después de amamantar.

LANGUAGE REVIEW: PRESENT TENSE

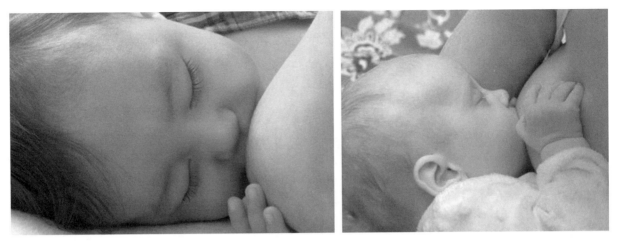

Exercise 6. Review the information on present tense conjugation from Chapter 2. Conjugate the verbs in the present tense in the following sentences to describe a nurse helping a new mother achieve an effective latch.

1. La enfermera _____ (ayudar) a la mamá a tener un buen enganche.

2. La mamá y la enfermera _____ (mirar) al bebé.

3. La bebé _____ (buscar) el pecho.

4. La bebé _____ (llevar) sólo el pañal.

5. La enfermera _____ (enseñar) a la mamá la posición de cuna.

🎧 LISTENING COMPREHENSION

Exercise 7. Listen to the dialogue on the audio file between a mother and a lactation consultant as they discuss milk supply; then answer the comprehension questions in English.

1. What did the mother want to know at the beginning of the conversation?

_____

2. How often did the lactation consultant suggest the mother feed the baby?

_____

3. What did the lactation consultant say about the milk production system?

_____

4. How often is the mother currently feeding her baby?

_____

Exercise 8. Breastfeeding Intake Exercise

In this exercise, you will listen to a conversation between a mother and a breastfeeding support person. The support person is gathering information about the mother and baby to complete an intake form. Listen to their conversation. Fill in the answers on the intake form in English.

Breastfeeding Intake Form

1. Mother's name　　　　　_____

2. Baby's name　　　　　　_____

3. Phone number　　　　　_____

4. Pediatrician　　　　　　_____

5. Baby's birthdate　　　　_____

6. Baby's birth weight　　　_____

7. Current weight　　　　　_____

8. Number of feedings in 24 hours　　_____

9. Formula use (yes/no)　　_____

10. Pacifier use (yes/no)　　_____

TEAR-OUT QUICK REFERENCE: MILK SUPPLY

KEY VOCABULARY	
ENGLISH	**SPANISH**
milk supply	cantidad de leche, producción de leche
feeding (breastfeeding)	toma, comida de pecho, lactada
foremilk	leche inicial
hindmilk	leche final
breastpump	sacaleches, bomba, tiraleches
to pump milk	sacarse la leche, extraer la leche

SABER		CONOCER	
To know a fact or information	**Sabemos** que es importante evitar la formula. *[We know it is important to avoid formula.]*	**To be familiar with a place**	**Conozco** el hospital. *[I'm familiar with the hospital.]*
	No **sé** si estoy produciendo suficiente leche. *[I don't know whether I am producing enough milk.]*	**To be familiar or know a person**	Ella **conoce** a la consultora de lactancia. *[She knows the lactation consultant.]* No **conocemos** al doctor. *[We do not know the doctor.]*
	No **sé** cómo usar la posición de cuna cruzada. *[I don't know how to use the cross-cradle hold.]*	**To be familiar with a concept**	Las madres **conocen** la técnica de alimentar a demanda. *[The mothers are familiar with the technique of cue feeding.]*

COMMON PHRASES	
ENGLISH	**SPANISH**
Let's see…	Vamos a ver…
I think you should…	Creo que debería…
To stop using it	Dejar de usarlo
It's a supply and demand system.	Es un sistema de oferta y demanda.
Pumping after feedings increases milk supply.	Extraer la leche después de dar pecho aumenta la producción de leche.
I recommend using a hospital grade pump.	Recomiendo usar un sacaleches de calidad de hospital.
You can rent one here.	Puede alquilar uno aquí.
I recommend leaving the baby on the first breast until he falls asleep or comes off the breast.	Recomiendo dejar al bebé en el primer pecho hasta que se duerma o él sólo se retire.

Notes for the Classroom Instructor

This section is for instructors using this book in a classroom setting.

Section A: Present Progressive

A good exercise to practice the present progressive is to show the students a series of pictures (images taken from magazines or books) and have them describe what is going on in each in the immediate present.

Section B: *Saber/Conocer*

1. Although these two words are taught together, it may be better to practice them separately in order to reinforce the difference in their meanings in Spanish. If you have supplementary exercises or worksheets, try to focus on one word at a time.

2. A good classroom activity for *conocer* is to ask students if they are familiar with certain places and ask them to describe these places (San Francisco, Chicago, New York). These types of exercises can incorporate adjectives as well.

3. You will also want to explain the personal *a* in Spanish in connection with the verb *conocer* (see below). Students can ask each other whether they have ever met a celebrity or if they know people with certain characteristics.

A note about the "personal *a*": The use of the word *a* before a person who is a direct object in the sentence is frequently taught in Spanish textbooks.

Examples:

• Voy a llamar **a** la doctora.

• Voy a llamar **al** doctor.

• Alimento **a** la bebé cada dos horas.

• La consejera de lactancia ayuda **a** las madres.

While it is helpful to understand the placement of this preposition and absolutely necessary to textbook-correct Spanish, the authors have chosen to omit a discussion of it in the self-teaching modules because of its relative unimportance in learning to communicate in Spanish. However, it may be appropriate for a classroom explanation.

ANSWER KEY

Need help with these exercises? Looking for more opportunities to practice? For support and additional resources to help you learn to provide breastfeeding support in Spanish, visit www.spanishforbreastfeedingsupport.com.

Exercise 1.

1. no está creciendo bien

2. por la cantidad de peso que aumenta y el número de pañales mojados y sucios

3. cada tres horas, a veces cada cuatro horas de noche

4. de un sistema de oferta y demanda

5. Any two of the following: alimentar al bebé con frecuencia, cada dos a tres horas, ofrecer al bebé los dos pechos, apretar el pecho durante la alimentación, extraer la leche después de alimentar al bebé, hierbas y alimentos, tener un buen enganche

Exercise 2.

1. está amamantando *[She is breastfeeding her three-day-old baby.]*

2. está sosteniendo *[Claudia is holding the baby skin-to-skin.]*

3. están ayudando *[The lactation consultants are helping Claudia find a good position.]*

4. está comiendo *[The baby is eating enough milk and Claudia…]*

5. está escuchando *[…is hearing a sound when Ricardo eats.]*

Exercise 3.

1. saben *[Mothers know that babies need to eat at least eight to 12 times every 24 hours.]*

2. conozco *[I don't know the lactation counselor.]*

3. conocemos *[We know many techniques to produce enough milk.]*

4. sabe *[She does not know what "skin-to-skin" means.]*

5. conoce *[Do you know the technique of feeding on cue?]*

Exercise 4.

1. conocemos *[We know a lactation counselor who can help you.]*

2. sabe *[The lactation counselor knows how to help mothers with sore nipples.]*

3. conocen *[The nurses know techniques for a good milk supply.]*

4. sé *[I do not know what "feeding on cue" means.]*

5. conoce *[She does not know the doctor.]*

Exercise 5. Can be any of these, in any order:
• Trate de
• Recomiendo
• Usted puede
• Creo que debería

Exercise 6.

1. ayuda *[The nurse helps the mother have a good latch.]*

2. miran *[The nurse and the mother look at the baby.]*

3. busca *[The baby looks for the breast.]*

4. lleva *[The baby wears only a diaper.]*

5. enseña *[The nurse shows the mother the cradle hold.]*

Listening Comprehension Dialogue:

Mother: ¿Con qué frecuencia debo alimentar al bebé?
[How often should I feed my baby?]

LC: La mayoría de los bebés necesitan comer al menos ocho a 12 veces en 24 horas.
[Most babies need to eat at least eight to 12 times in 24 hours.]

Mother: Entonces, ¿si amamanto mucho, produzco más leche?
[If I feed her often, will I make more milk?]

LC: Sí, es un sistema de oferta y demanda. ¿Con qué frecuencia está alimentando al bebé?
[Yes, it's a supply and demand system. How often are you feeding the baby?]

Mother: Le estoy dando pecho más o menos cada tres horas, a veces cada cuatro horas de noche.
[I'm feeding him about every three hours, sometimes every four hours at night.]

Exercise 7.

1. how frequently should she feed her baby

2. at least eight to 12 times in 24 hours

3. It is a supply and demand system.

4. every three hours, sometimes every four hours at night

Intake Dialogue

Q: ¿Cómo se llama?
A: Me llamo Teresa Salcedo.

Q: ¿Cómo se llama su bebé?
A: Se llama Daniel Mendoza.

Q: ¿Cuál es su número de teléfono?
A: Es el (212) 865-0505.

Q: ¿Cómo se llama el doctor de su bebé?
A: Se llama la doctora Sandoval.

Q: ¿Cuándo nació su bebé?
A: El seis de junio.

Q: ¿Cuánto pesó el bebé al nacer?
A: Pesó cinco libras con tres onzas.

Q: ¿Cuánto pesa su bebé ahora?
A: Pesa siete libras con 10 onzas.

Q: ¿Cuántas veces alimenta al bebé en 24 horas?
A: Más o menos 10 veces.

Q: ¿El bebé toma fórmula?
A: No, no uso fórmula.

Q: ¿Está usando un chupón?
A: A veces sí.

Exercise 8.

1. Mother's name: Teresa Salcedo

2. Baby's name: Daniel Mendoza

3. Phone number: (212) 865-0505

4. Pediatrician: Doctora Sandoval

5. Baby's birthdate: June 6

6. Baby's birth weight: 5 lbs., 3 ozs.

7. Current weight: 7 lbs, 10 ozs.

8. Number of feedings in 24 hours: 10

9. Formula use: no

10. Pacifier use: yes, sometimes

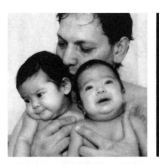

CHAPTER 6
INFANT GROWTH PATTERNS AND WEIGHT GAIN

OBJECTIVES

By the end of this chapter, you will be able to:

• Understand and use vocabulary and phrases related to infant growth patterns and weight gain

• Use expressions with the word *tener*

• Describe actions using adverbs

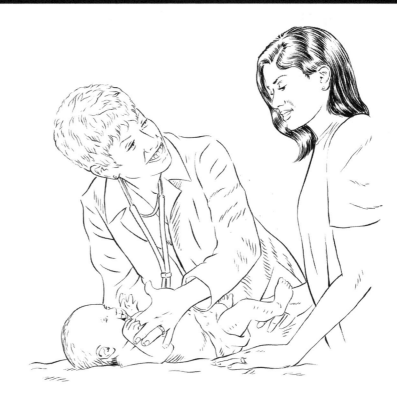

DIALOGUE

In this dialogue, a pediatrician discusses infant weight gain with the mother of a three-month-old baby. Listen to the dialogue as you read along in the book. Repeat each line, pausing the audio as necessary; then listen to the vocabulary and important phrases, and repeat each one.

Setting:
• **Pediatrician's office**

Characters:
• **Doctor (Dr. Wong)**
• **Mother (María)**
• **3-month-old baby**

Doctor: ¡Hola, María! Mire qué grande está su bebé!
    [Hi María! Look how big your baby is!]

Mother: Sí, está subiendo de peso. ¿Tiene un crecimiento normal?
    [Yes, she's getting bigger. Is she growing normally?]

NOTES

Doctor: Bueno, de acuerdo con el expediente, ella pesa 10 onzas más que la semana pasada. Ahora pesa 13 libras con dos onzas.
[Well, according to her chart she weighs 10 ounces more than last week. She now weighs 13 pounds, two ounces.]

Mother: ¿Eso está bien?
[Is that good?]

Doctor: ¡Sí, es excelente!
[Yes, it's great!]

Mother: ¿Cuánto aumentan los bebés normalmente?
[How much do babies usually gain?]

Doctor: Los bebés normalmente aumentan una onza por día, o aproximadamente cinco a ocho onzas por semana, durante los primeros tres meses. Aumentan de peso más lentamente después.
[Babies usually gain about an ounce a day, or about five to eight ounces a week, for the first three months. They gain more slowly after that.]

Mother: ¿Cómo puedo saber si mi bebé recibe suficiente leche?
[How can I tell if my baby's getting enough milk?]

Doctor: Se sabe por la cantidad de peso que aumenta y el número de pañales mojados y sucios.
[You can tell by the amount of weight she gains and the number of wet and dirty diapers she has.]

Mother: Hoy está comiendo tanto. Me preocupa que no reciba suficiente leche.
[She's eating so much today. I'm worried that she's not getting enough milk.]

Doctor: Posiblemente sea un estirón. Durante un estirón, los bebés comen con mucha frecuencia para aumentar la cantidad de leche que usted produce.
[Maybe it is a growth spurt. During a growth spurt, babies eat very often in order to increase your supply.]

Mother: Ya veo. ¿Tengo que introducir los alimentos sólidos pronto?
[I see. Do I have to start solid foods soon?]

Doctor: No. Recomendamos la lactancia materna exclusiva por los primeros seis meses.
[No. We recommend exclusive breastfeeding for the first six months.]

Mother: Y, ¿después de eso?
[And after that?]

Doctor: Recomendamos la introducción de alimentos sólidos a los seis meses, y la continuación de la lactancia materna durante por lo menos un año, y después del año por el tiempo que deseen la madre y el bebé.
[We recommend introducing solid foods at six months and continuing breastfeeding for at least one year, and as long after that as you and the baby want.]

Mother: Así que, ¿debo seguir alimentándola a demanda?
[So, I should go on nursing her on cue?]

Doctor: ¡Correcto! ¡Lo está haciendo muy bien!
[That's right! You're doing a great job!]

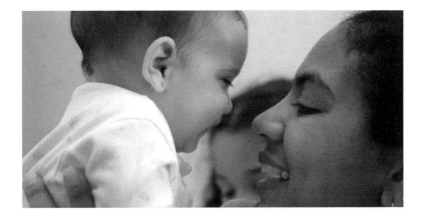

IMPORTANT PHRASES

1. Tener que...to have to (do something)

2. Tener cinco meses ....to be five months old

3. A esta edad... at this age

4. Lo está haciendo muy bien.............................. You're doing a great job.

COMPREHENSION QUESTIONS

Exercise 1. After reading and listening to the dialogue on the audio file, listen again without the text and answer the following questions in Spanish. Don't worry about forming complete sentences; simply focus on writing down the key information.

Note: If you are completing the exercises in this chapter for CERPs, write your answers on the answer sheets provided in Appendix A.

1. What is María concerned about?

_____

2. How many ounces did María's baby gain this week?

_____

3. What does the doctor say about how much weight babies usually gain during the first three months?

_____

4. What does the doctor say happens during a growth spurt?

_____

5. What does the doctor say about when babies should begin solid foods?

_____

VOCABULARY

1. alimentos sólidos...................solid foods

2. año...year

3. aproximadamente.............approximately

4. cantidad....................................amount

5. crecimiento....................................growth

6. de acuerdo con..........in accordance with, according to

7. día..day

8. en..at, in

9. estirón.............................. growth spurt

10. exclusivo/a .... exclusive

11. expediente .... chart, file

12. hasta...until

13. lentamente................................. slowly

14. listo...ready

15. más que...................................more than

16. mes ....month

17. mojado ....wet

18. noche ....night

19. normalmente ....normally

20. número ....number

21. peso .... weight

22. primero.. first

23. probablemente...................... probably

24. pronto..soon

25. seguir................................ to continue

26. subir de peso.................. to gain weight

27. sucio.. dirty

LANGUAGE LESSONS

A. *TENER* EXPRESSIONS

In Spanish, the verb *tener* means "to have." *Tener* is used to express several concepts that are important for breastfeeding support, such as age, hunger, thirst, and having to do something. Let's begin by looking at the conjugation of *tener* in the present tense, which is irregular in the *yo* form and has a spelling change in other forms.

TENER	
Yo: **Tengo**	Nosotros: **Tenemos**
Tú: **Tienes**	
Él, Ella, Usted: **Tienen**	Ellos, Ustedes: **Tienen**

TENER TO EXPRESS AGE

Instead of saying that the baby **is** 2 months old, in Spanish we say that the baby **has** (*tiene*) 2 months.

Examples:

- Mi bebé **tiene** seis meses. *[My baby is six months old.]*
- Yo **tengo** 34 años. *[I am 34 years old.]*

TENER TO EXPRESS PHYSICAL AND MENTAL STATES

Instead of saying that the baby **is** hungry, in Spanish we say that the baby **has** (*tiene*) hunger. This also applies to the following physical and mental states:

TENER EXPRESSIONS	
Tener hambre	To be hungry
Tener sed	To be thirsty
Tener frío	To be cold
Tener calor	To be hot
Tener miedo	To be afraid
Tener prisa	To be in a hurry
Tener razón	To be right
Tener sueño	To be sleepy

Examples:

- El bebé **tiene hambre** cada dos horas. *[The baby is hungry every two hours.]*
- A veces, los bebés **tienen sueño** después de comer. *[Sometimes, babies are sleepy after eating.]*

Exercise 2. Write three *tener* expressions for each of the persons described below, first indicating the age of the person, and then two mental or physical conditions drawn from the list on the previous page.

Example: male baby, three months old

- El bebé tiene tres meses.
- El bebé tiene hambre.
- El bebé tiene frío.

1. female baby, two weeks old

_____

_____

_____

2. mother, twenty-eight years old

_____

_____

_____

3. male baby, four months old

_____

_____

_____

TENER TO EXPRESS HAVING TO DO SOMETHING

In order to express "to have to" do something in Spanish, we pair *tener* with *que* and put it in front of an unconjugated verb. Here are some examples:

- Las madres **tienen que alimentar** a los bebés cada dos a tres horas.
[Mothers have to feed their babies every two to three hours.]

- Algunos bebés **tienen que comer** con más frecuencia.
[Some babies have to eat more frequently.]

Exercise 3. Write three basic instructions for positioning, using *tener que* plus the unconjugated verb.

Example: (alimentar) *Tiene que alimentar* al bebé cada dos horas.

1. (comenzar) _____

2. (poner) _____

3. (sostener) _____

B. DESCRIBING ACTION WORDS (ADVERBS)

Adverbs describe action words (verbs). There are some examples of adverbs in the introductory dialogue (normally, slowly). Just as in English, adverbs in Spanish are formed by modifying an adjective (for example, "normal" becomes "normally").

You learned in Chapter 4 that most adjectives either end in **–o** or **–a**, depending on the gender of the word they describe. However, there are some adjectives ending in **–e** or in a consonant, which do not change according to gender.

For those adjectives ending in **–o** or **–a**, the adverb is formed by making the adjective feminine (ending with **–a**) and adding the ending *–mente*. For example:

Rápido   ⟶   rápida   ⟶   rápida*mente [quickly]*

Lento   ⟶   lenta   ⟶   lenta*mente [slowly]*

For those adjectives that end in **–e** or a consonant, the spelling of the adjective remains the same, and *–mente* is added to form the adverb. Example:

Feliz   ⟶   feliz*mente [happily]*

Triste   ⟶   triste*mente [sadly]*

Exercise 4. Change the adjectives in parentheses into adverbs to describe the action word in each sentence.

1. El bebé come _____ (lento).

2. El bebé termina con un pecho _____ (rápido).

3. Después de comer, el bebé _____duerme (normal).

LANGUAGE REVIEW: *SER/ESTAR*

Exercise 5. Review the uses of *ser* and *estar* in Chapter 4. Decide which of the two verbs to use in the following sentences, and conjugate them in the present tense.

1. La enfermera _____ de Puerto Rico.

2. Los bebés _____ felices cuando comen con frecuencia.

3. Nosotros _____ en la clínica todos los días de la semana.

4. Yo _____ cansada porque mi bebé come mucho.

5. Ella _____ consultora de lactancia.

LISTENING COMPREHENSION

Exercise 6. Listen to the dialogue on the audio file between a mother and a pediatrician as they discuss infant growth and weight gain; then answer the comprehension questions in English.

1. What did the mother ask the doctor about her baby?

_____

2. What did the doctor say about her baby's weight gain?

_____

3. What did the doctor say about normal growth at this age?

_____

4. When does the doctor advise starting solid foods?

_____

Exercise 7. Breastfeeding Intake Exercise

In this exercise, you will listen to a conversation between a mother and a breastfeeding support person. The support person is gathering information about the mother and baby to complete an intake form. Listen to their conversation. Fill in the answers on the intake form in English.

Breastfeeding Intake Form

1. Mother's name _____

2. Baby's name _____

3. Phone number _____

4. Pediatrician _____

5. Baby's birthdate _____

6. Baby's birth weight _____

7. Current weight _____

8. Number of feedings in 24 hours _____

9. Number of wet diapers in 24 hours _____

10. Number of dirty diapers in 24 hours _____

11. Color of dirty diapers _____

12. Formula use (yes/no) _____

13. Pacifier use (yes/no) _____

Tear-Out Quick Reference: Infant Growth Patterns and Weight Gain

KEY VOCABULARY	
ENGLISH	**SPANISH**
solid foods	alimentos sólidos
to gain weight	aumentar
to grow	crecer
growth spurt	estirón
ounces	onzas

COMMON *TENER* EXPRESSIONS	
ENGLISH	**SPANISH**
To be hungry	Tener hambre
To be thirsty	Tener sed
To be cold	Tener frío
To be hot	Tener calor
To be afraid	Tener miedo
To be in a hurry	Tener prisa
To be right	Tener razón
To be sleepy	Tener sueño
To be _____ years (months) old	Tener _____ años (meses)
To have to…	Tener que…

COMMON ADVERBS	
ENGLISH	**SPANISH**
quickly	rápidamente
slowly	lentamente
happily	felizmente
normally	normalmente
sadly	tristemente

COMMON PHRASES AND QUESTIONS	
ENGLISH	**SPANISH**
The baby weighs _____ pounds.	El bebé pesa _____ libras.
He/she is growing normally.	Tiene un crecimiento normal.
Babies usually gain about an ounce a day, or around 5 to 8 ounces a week, until they are about three months old.	Los bebés normalmente ganan una onza por día, o aproximadamente 5 a 8 onzas por semana, hasta los tres meses.
During a growth spurt, babies eat very often in order to increase your supply.	Durante un estirón, los bebés comen con mucha frecuencia para aumentar la cantidad de leche que usted produce.
You should keep feeding her on cue.	Debe seguir alimentándola a demanda.
You're doing a great job.	Lo está haciendo muy bien.

Notes for the Classroom Instructor

This section is for instructors using this book in a classroom setting.

Section A: *Tener* expressions

The teacher can make use of visuals to teach the various uses of *tener*, particularly the physical and mental states. One activity is to tear out a variety of pictures and images from magazines and ask students to describe the people in the pictures, using *tener* expressions. The students can guess the person's age and make comments related to the person being cold, sleepy, hot, or fearful. Students can do this kind of activity in pairs with a single picture that is then presented to the class, or the teacher can hold up images to the group as a whole and have them work together to describe the people in them.

Section B: Adverbs

Just as you showed students action pictures to practice forming the present progressive in Chapter 5, you can take that exercise a step further and ask them to use adverbs to more precisely describe the actions they observe.

ANSWER KEY

Need help with these exercises? Looking for more opportunities to practice? For support and additional resources to help you learn to provide breastfeeding support in Spanish, visit www.spanishforbreastfeedingsupport.com.

Exercise 1.

1. si tiene un crecimiento normal

2. diez onzas

3. una onza por día, o aproximadamente cinco a ocho onzas por semana

4. durante un estirón, los bebés comen con mucha frecuencia para aumentar la cantidad de leche que usted produce

5. a los seis meses, aproximadamente

Exercise 2. Answers will vary after the first sentence, but may include:

1. la bebé tiene dos semanas, tiene hambre, tiene sueño

2. la madre tiene veintiocho años, tiene sueño, tiene prisa

3. el bebé tiene cuatro meses, tiene sed, tiene frío

Exercise 3. Answers will vary, but may include sentences similar to the following:

1. Tiene que comenzar con el bebé piel con piel contra su pecho. *[You have to start with the baby skin-to-skin against your chest.]*

2. Tiene que poner la mano en su espalda y los hombros. *[You have to place your hand on his back and shoulders.]*

3. Tiene que sostener el pecho con la otra mano. *[You have to hold your breast with your other hand.]*

Exercise 4.

1. lentamente *[The baby eats slowly.]*

2. rápidamente *[The baby finishes with one breast quickly.]*

3. normalmente *[After eating, the baby normally sleeps.]*

Exercise 5.

1. es *[The nurse is from Puerto Rico.]*

2. están *[The babies are happy when they eat frequently.]*

3. estamos *[We are in the clinic every day of the week.]*

4. estoy *[I am tired because my baby eats a lot.]*

5. es *[She is a lactation counselor.]*

Listening Comprehension Dialogue:

Mother: Hola, doctor. ¿Mi bebé está creciendo bien? *[Hi, Doctor. Do you think my baby is growing well?]*

Doctor: Sí, está aumentando de peso bien. *[Yes, he is gaining weight well.]*

Mother: ¿Cuánto debe aumentar el bebé en una semana? *[How much should my baby gain in one week?]*

Doctor: Los bebés normalmente aumentan una onza por día a esta edad. *[Babies usually gain about an ounce a day at this age.]*

Mother: OK. Y, ¿cuándo debo introducir alimentos sólidos? *[Okay. And when should I start solid foods?]*

Doctor: Puede introducir alimentos sólidos cuando el bebé tiene seis meses. *[You can start solids when your baby is six months old.]*

Exercise 6.

1. If her baby is growing well

2. He is gaining weight well.

3. Normally, babies gain one ounce per day.

4. When he is six months old

Breastfeeding Intake Dialogue

Q: Hola. ¿Cómo se llama?
A: Me llamo Catalina Hernández.

Q: ¿Cómo se llama su bebé?
A: Se llama Diego Hernández.

Q: ¿Cuál es su número de teléfono?
A: Es el (823) 219-7453.

Q: ¿Cómo se llama el doctor de su bebé?
A: Se llama el doctor Salas.

Q: ¿Cuándo nació su bebé?
A: El veinticuatro de mayo.

Q: ¿Cuánto pesó el bebé al nacer?
A: Pesó siete libras con dos onzas.

Q: ¿Cuánto pesa su bebé ahora?
A: Ahora pesa siete libras con diez onzas.

Q: ¿Cuántas veces alimenta al bebé en 24 horas?
A: 9 o 10 veces.

Q: ¿Cuántos pañales mojados hace el bebé en 24 horas?
A: Más o menos 9.

Q: ¿Cuántos pañales sucios hace el bebé en 24 horas?
A: Creo que 5.

Q: ¿De qué color son los pañales sucios del bebé?
A: Son de color amarillo-anaranjado.

Q: ¿El bebé toma fórmula?
A: No.

Q: ¿El bebé usa un chupón?
A: Sí, a veces.

Exercise 7.

1. Mother's name: Catalina Hernández

2. Baby's name: Diego Hernández

3. Phone number: (823) 219-7453

4. Pediatrician: Dr. Salas

5. Baby's birthdate: May 24

6. Baby's birth weight: 7 lbs., 2 ozs.

7. Current weight: 7 lbs., 10 ozs.

8. Number of feedings in 24 hours: 9-10 times

9. Number of wet diapers in 24 hours: about 9

10. Number of dirty diapers in 24 hours: 5

11. Color of dirty diapers: yellow-orange

12. Formula use (yes/no): no

13. Pacifier use (yes/no): yes

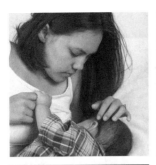

CHAPTER 7
COMMON BREASTFEEDING CHALLENGES

OBJECTIVES

By the end of this chapter, you will be able to:

• Understand and use vocabulary and phrases related to common breastfeeding challenges

• Use *ir* + *a* to express future plans

• Express possession or ownership

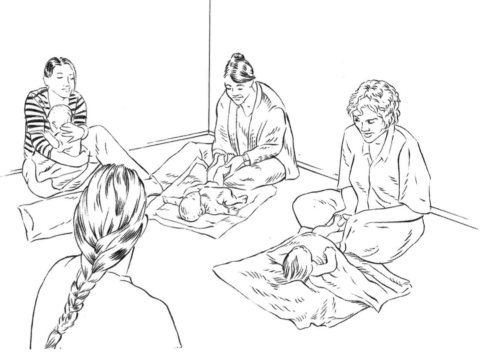

🎧 DIALOGUE

In this dialogue, three mothers are discussing breastfeeding challenges with a breastfeeding support group leader. Listen to the dialogue as you read along in the book. Repeat each line, pausing the audio as necessary; then listen to the vocabulary and important phrases, and repeat each one.

Setting:
• **Breastfeeding support group**

Characters:
• **Group leader**
• **Several mothers**

Leader: ¡Bienvenidas todas! Vamos a hablar de cómo les va con la lactancia.
    [Greetings everyone! We're going to talk about how breastfeeding is going for you.]

Mother 1: Bueno, la semana pasada estaba muy hinchada.
    [Well, last week I was very engorged.]

Leader: ¿Qué hacen ustedes cuando están hinchadas?
    [What do you all do when you are engorged?]

Mother 2: El doctor dice que tengo que alimentar mucho a mi bebé. Uso compresas frías en los pechos después de amamantar y extraigo un poco de leche. Mi hermana usa hojas de col en sus pechos.
[The doctor says that I have to feed my baby a lot. I use cold compresses on my breasts after feedings and express a little milk. My sister uses cabbage leaves on her breasts.]

Leader: Sus soluciones son muy buenas. ¿Y usted?
[Your solutions are very good. How about you?]

Mother 3: Estoy preocupada porque siento un bulto en el seno. Creo que es un conducto lácteo obstruido.
[I'm worried because I feel a hard spot in my breast. I think it's a plugged duct.]

Leader: Lo siento mucho. ¿Dónde le duele?
[I'm sorry to hear that. Where does it hurt?]

Mother 3: Me duele aquí.
[It hurts right here.]

Leader: Cuando amamante, masajee esa área suavemente, y cambie de posiciones frecuentemente. También puede utilizar una compresa mojada con agua caliente antes de amamantar o extraer la leche.
[When you nurse, massage that area gently, and change positions frequently. You can also use a warm, wet compress before nursing or pumping.]

Mother 3: ¿Está infectado?
[Is it infected?]

Leader: A veces los conductos obstruidos se infectan. Eso se llama mastitis. Si tiene síntomas de la gripe—fiebre, escalofríos, dolores—llame a su doctor.
[Sometimes plugged ducts get infected. That's called mastitis. If you have symptoms of the flu – fever, chills, aches - call your doctor.]

Mother 3: Si está infectado, ¿qué tengo que hacer?
[If it's infected, what do I have to do?]

Leader: Siga amamantando en ese pecho, descanse mucho y tome mucho líquido. Su doctor posiblemente le dé antibióticos.
[Continue to nurse on that breast, and get plenty of rest and fluids. Your doctor may give you antibiotics.]

Mother 1: El bebé de mi hermana tiene una infección de hongo. ¿Cómo puedo saber si tengo algo así?
[My sister's baby has thrush. How can I tell if I have something like that?]

Leader: Una infección de hongo causa un ardor durante la lactancia, y su bebé puede tener unas manchas blancas en la boca que no se quitan. Posiblemente necesite medicamentos.
[Thrush causes a burning pain when you nurse, and your baby might have some white patches in her mouth that don't rub off. You may need medication.]

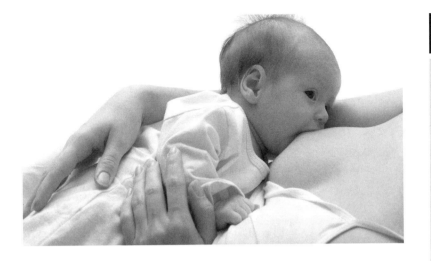

IMPORTANT PHRASES

1. Vamos a intentar...Let's try.

2. Estaba muy hinchada ....I was very engorged.

3. Llame a su doctor...Call your doctor.

COMPREHENSION QUESTIONS

Exercise 1. After reading and listening to the dialogue on the audio file, listen again without the text and answer the following questions in Spanish. Don't worry about forming complete sentences; simply focus on writing down the key information.

Note: If you are completing the exercises in this chapter for CERPs, write your answers on the answer sheets provided in Appendix A.

1. What is Mother #1's breastfeeding challenge?

_____

2. What can Mother #1 do to manage this issue?

_____

3. What is Mother #3 worried about?

_____

4. When should Mother #3 call the doctor?

_____

5. What does the support group leader say are signs of thrush?

_____

VOCABULARY

1. antibióticos ....antibiotics

2. aquí..here

3. ardor..burning sensation

4. área... area

5. bienvenidos/as ....welcome

6. bulto...lump, mass

7. compresa caliente .... warm compress

8. compresa fría.............................cold compress

9. compresa mojada..........................wet compress

10. conducto lácteo obstruido ....plugged duct

11. dolores...aches, pains

12. escalofríos.. chills

13. fiebre...fever

14. gripe...flu, cold

15. hablar.................................to talk, to speak

16. hermana...sister

17. hinchado/a ....engorged, swollen

18. hojas de col .... cabbage leaves

19. infección de hongo, algodoncillo .... thrush

20. infectado..infected

21. líquidos ....fluids, liquids

22. mancha... spot

23. masajear..to massage

24. mastitis .... mastitis

25. muy.. very

26. reto.. challenge

27. síntomas...symptoms

28. solución...solution

29. suavemente ....gently

30. utilizar ....to use

LANGUAGE LESSONS

A. TALKING ABOUT THE FUTURE

One way to say that you are "going to do" something in the future is to conjugate the verb *ir* ("to go") in the present tense, and follow it with *a* and an unconjugated verb.

First, let's review the conjugation of the verb *ir*:

IR	
Yo: **Voy**	Nosotros: **Vamos**
Tú: **Vas**	
Él, Ella, Usted: **Va**	Ellos, Ustedes: **Van**

After conjugating *ir* according to the person who is going to do something, we add *a* plus an unconjugated verb to make the following construction:

ir + *a* + **unconjugated verb**

Examples:

• Ella **va a usar** una compresa fría si está hinchada.
[She is going to use a cold compress if she is engorged.]

• Si ella tiene fiebre y escalofríos, **va a llamar** al doctor.
[If she has fever and chills, she is going to call the doctor.]

Exercise 2. Use an *ir* + *a* expression to fill in the blanks, as in the following example:

Sofía _____ (extraer) un poco de leche con el sacaleches después de amamantar al bebé.

Sofía **va a extraer** un poco de leche con el sacaleches después de amamantar al bebé.

1. Las madres _____(tener) muchas preguntas acerca de retos comunes de la lactancia.

2. El doctor le _____ (dar) un antibiótico si tiene mastitis.

3. Si tiene una infección, Carolina _____ (alimentar) al bebé mucho, tomar antibióticos, descansar y tomar mucho líquido.

4. Yo _____(usar) hojas de col para el hinchazón.

5. Usted _____ (sentir) un ardor cuando da pecho si tiene una infección de hongo.

B. EXPRESSING POSSESSION

The following words are used to express possession in Spanish:

POSSESSIVE ADJECTIVES	
My: **mi/mis**	Our: **nuestro/nuestra/nuestros/ nuestras**
Your: **tu/tus**	
His, Her, Your (formal): **su/sus**	Their, Your (formal): **su/sus**

Because these words are adjectives, they will "agree" in number (singular or plural) with the object(s) or person(s) they describe. In the case of "our," the possessive adjective will also agree in gender. See the examples below:

- **Mi esposo** se llama Samuel.
[My husband is named Samuel.]

- **Sus pechos** están hinchados.
[Her breasts are engorged.]

- **Nuestras enfermeras** pueden ayudar con la lactancia.
[Our nurses can help with breastfeeding.]

Exercise 3. Translate the possessive adjectives in the following sentences, making sure they agree with the word they describe in number and gender.

Estoy en un grupo de apoyo a la lactancia. _____ (my) amiga, Jessica, también está en el grupo. Llevamos a _____ (our) bebés al grupo para hablar de los retos de la lactancia. Esta semana Jessica siente un bulto en el pecho. La líder del grupo dice que Jessica posiblemente tenga un conducto lácteo obstruido. Las otras madres en el grupo hacen recomendaciones, como compresas calientes y masajes en el pecho. Si tiene síntomas de gripe, Jessica debe llamar a _____ (her) doctor inmediatemente. Estoy muy feliz con mi grupo de apoyo. Las otras madres me ayudan con _____ (my) problemas con la lactancia y hablamos de _____ (our) triunfos (triumphs) también.

C. Pronunciation Practice

The Spanish language does not distinguish between the sounds for *b* and *v*—they are both equivalent to the b sound in English. In other words, there is no distinct *v* sound in Spanish.

However, the *b/v* sound in Spanish has two variations: hard and soft. The hard *b* sound is used when the *b* or *v* is the first letter of the word or follows the letters m or n. The hard *b* is formed with the lips together, just like a *b* sound in English. It is made when pronouncing the various conjugations of the frequently used verb *ir: voy, vas, va, vamos, van*. With the hard *b*, these words will sound like "*boy, bas, ba, bamos, ban.*"

When the *b* or *v* is in the middle of a word (except after m or n), it has a softer pronunciation, and the lips do not meet. Examples of the softer *b* sound in Spanish words are: *fiebre, abuela, labios*.

Tongue Twisters (Trabalenguas). Listen to the tongue twisters on the audio file, making note of the slightly different pronunciations of the *b* sound, then repeat after the speaker and try to keep up!

1. Estaba en el bosque Francisco buscando al obispo vasco, y al verlo le dijo al obispo: "Busco al obispo vasco."
[Francisco was in the forest looking for the Basque bishop, and when he saw him, he said to the bishop: "I'm looking for the Basque bishop."]

2. Barre con la escoba, boba, y no barras con la vara, que la vara no es escoba.
[Sweep with the broom, silly, and don't sweep with the wand, because the wand is not a broom.]

Language Review: Greetings

Exercise 4. Review the lesson on greetings from Chapter 1 and the ways in which the different characters have greeted each other in the dialogues you have read and heard; then organize the following six statements and questions into a conversation.

a. Mucho gusto, Ana. Me llamo Celia.

b. ¿Cómo le va con la lactancia hoy?

c. Buenos días. Me llamo Ana.

d. Me va bien, gracias.

e. Estoy bien.

f. Mucho gusto, Celia. ¿Cómo está?

1. _____

2. _____

3. _____

4. _____

5. _____

6. _____

 ## LISTENING COMPREHENSION

Exercise 5. Listen to the dialogue on the audio file between a mother and a breastfeeding support group leader as they discuss mastitis; then answer the comprehension questions in English.

1. Why is the mother worried?

_____

2. What symptoms does she have?

_____

3. What does the support group leader suggest she do?

_____

4. What other advice does the support group leader have?

_____

5. Who will help the mother so she can rest?

_____

Tear-Out Quick Reference: Common Breastfeeding Challenges

KEY VOCABULARY	
ENGLISH	**SPANISH**
thrush	infección de hongo, algodoncillo
plugged duct	conducto lácteo obstruido
infection	infección
lump, hard spot on the breast	bulto en el pecho
fever	fiebre
chills	escalofríos
body aches	dolores del cuerpo
antibiotic	antibiótico
compress (cold or hot)	compresa (fría o caliente)
to rest	descansar
mastitis	mastitis
cabbage leaves	hojas de col

EXPRESSING FUTURE PLANS	
IR **+** A **+** UNCONJUGATED VERB	
I am going to call the doctor.	Voy a llamar al doctor.
She is going to use a cold compress.	Ella va a utilizar una compresa fría.
The doctor is going to give you an antibiotic.	El doctor le va a dar un antibiótico.
We are going to try a new position.	Vamos a intentar otra posición.

POSSESSIVE ADJECTIVES	
My: **mi/mis**	Our: **nuestro/nuestra/nuestros/nuestras**
Your: **tu/tus**	
His, Her, Your (formal): **su/sus**	Their, Your (formal): **su/sus**

COMMON PHRASES	
ENGLISH	**SPANISH**
Where does it hurt?	¿Dónde le duele?
Massage that area gently.	Masajee esa área suavemente.
Do you have fever, chills, or body aches?	¿Tiene fiebre, escalofríos o dolores del cuerpo?
Continue to nurse on that breast, get lots of rest and drink a lot of fluids.	Siga amamantando en ese pecho, descanse mucho y tome mucho líquido.
Use cold compresses on your breasts after feedings.	Use compresas frías en sus pechos después de amamantar.
Thrush causes a burning pain when you nurse, and your baby might have some white patches in her mouth that don't rub off.	Una infección de hongo causa un ardor durante la lactancia, y su bebé puede tener unas manchas blancas en la boca que no se quitan.

Notes for the Classroom Instructor

This section is for instructors using this book in a classroom setting.

Section A: *Ir + a* expressions

The *ir + a* structure is very handy for first-time language learners because it allows them to express something that will happen in the future without having to learn another tense. Once they are able to memorize the proper conjugation of *ir*, it is easy to add on any infinitive to express a future plan. This lends itself to good classroom conversations. For example, you can ask each student to tell the class what he/she will do over the weekend. This can be a regular classroom conversation activity before each weekend.

Section B: Possessive Adjectives

The teacher can ask the students a series of questions beginning with "De quién es…" in order to practice the use of possessive adjectives. For example:

• "¿De quién es el salón de clases?" Answer: Es nuestro salón de clases.

• "¿De quién es el libro?" Answer: Es su libro. Or: Es mi libro.

Answer Key

Need help with these exercises? Looking for more opportunities to practice? For support and additional resources to help you learn to provide breastfeeding support in Spanish, visit www.spanishforbreastfeedingsupport.com.

Exercise 1.

1. cuando me bajó la leche estaba muy hinchada, hinchazón

2. alimentar mucho al bebé, compresas frías, extraer la leche, hojas de col

3. un bulto en el seno, conducto lácteo obstruido

4. si tiene síntomas de gripe: fiebre, escalofríos, dolores del cuerpo

5. ardor durante la lactancia, manchas blancas en la boca del bebé

Exercise 2.

1. van a tener *[The mothers are going to have a lot of questions about common breastfeeding challenges.]*

2. va a dar *[The doctor is going to give her an antibiotic if she has mastitis.]*

3. va a alimentar *[If she has an infection, Carolina is going to feed the baby a lot, take antibiotics, rest, and drink a lot of liquids.]*

4. voy a usar *[I am going to use cabbage leaves for engorgement.]*

5. va a sentir *[You are going to feel burning when you breastfeed if you have thrush.]*

Exercise 3.

1. Mi *[My friend, Jessica, is also in the group.]*

2. nuestros or nuestras *[We take our babies to the group to talk about breastfeeding challenges.]*

3. su *[If she has flu-like symptoms, Jessica should call her doctor immediately.]*

4. mis *[The other mothers help me with my breastfeeding problems...]*

5. nuestros *[...and we talk about our triumphs also.]*

Exercise 4.

1. c

2. a

3. f

4. e

5. b

6. d

Listening Comprehension Dialogue

Mother: Estoy preocupada porque creo que tengo una infección del pecho. Tengo una mancha roja en el pecho, y me duele. *[I'm worried because I think I have a breast infection. I have a red spot on my breast, and it hurts.]*

Leader: ¿Tiene fiebre, escalofríos o dolores del cuerpo? *[Do you have fever, chills, or aches?]*

Mother: Creo que tengo fiebre, y siento dolores en el cuerpo. *[I think I have a fever, and I feel achy.]*

Leader: Cuando tiene esos síntomas, llame al doctor. *[When you have those symptoms, call the doctor.]*

Mother: ¿Debo seguir amamantando de ese pecho? *[Should I keep nursing on that breast?]*

Leader: Sí, es importante seguir amamantando de ese pecho. También tiene que descansar y tomar mucho líquido. *[Yes, it's important to keep nursing*

on that breast. You also have to rest and drink a lot of liquids.]

Mother: OK. Creo que mi hermana puede ayudar con el bebé. ¿Tengo que tomar un medicamento? *[Okay, I think my sister can help me with the baby. Do I need to take a medication?]*

Leader: Su doctor probablemente le dé un antibiótico. *[Your doctor will probably give you an antibiotic.]*

Exercise 5.

1. she thinks she has an infection in her breast

2. a red spot on her breast, it hurts, fever and aches

3. to call the doctor

4. keep nursing on that breast, rest, drink lot of liquids

5. her sister

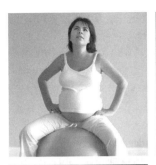

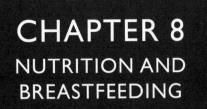

CHAPTER 8
NUTRITION AND BREASTFEEDING

OBJECTIVES

By the end of this chapter, you will be able to:

• Understand and use vocabulary and phrases related to nutrition and breastfeeding

• Discuss single occurrences in the past

• Use impersonal expressions

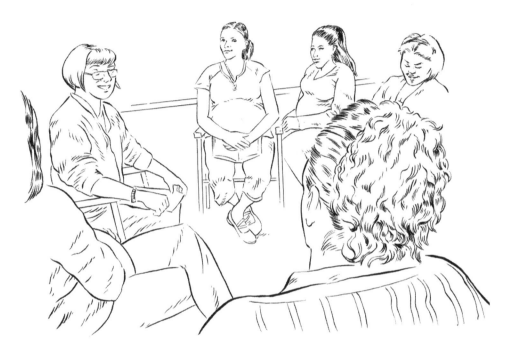

🎧 DIALOGUE

In this dialogue, a childbirth educator is discussing nutrition with women in a prenatal breastfeeding class. Listen to the dialogue as you read along in the book. Repeat each line, pausing the audio as necessary; then listen to the vocabulary and important phrases, and repeat each one.

Setting:
• **Prenatal breastfeeding class**

Characters:

• **Pregnant mothers**

• **Childbirth Educator (CE)**

CE: ¿Qué consejos han recibido acerca de lo que se debe comer durante la lactancia?
[Greetings everyone! What advice have you received about what to eat when you are breastfeeding?]

Mother 1: Mi hermana dijo que no se debe comer alimentos que causan gases. ¿Es cierto?
[My sister said that I shouldn't eat gassy foods. Is that true?]

CE: Muchos dicen eso. Pero cada bebé es diferente, y no hay ningún alimento que cause problemas a todos los bebés.
[Many people say that. But every baby is different, and there aren't any foods that upset all babies.]

Mother 1: ¿Así que puedo comer esos alimentos?
[So I can eat those foods?]

CE: Sí. Simplemente coma una buena dieta balanceada con muchas frutas, vegetales, granos y proteína. Si su bebé tiene una reacción a un alimento en su dieta, puede dejar de comerlo por un rato para ver si eso ayuda.
[Yes. Just eat a good, balanced diet with lots of fruit, vegetables, grains, and protein. If your baby reacts to something in your diet, you can stop eating it for a little while and see if it helps.]

Mother 1: Y, ¿el agua? ¿Es necesario tomar mucha agua para producir más leche?
[What about water? Do you have to drink a lot to make more milk?]

CE: No, simplemente tome agua cuando usted tenga sed.
[No, just drink to your thirst.]

Mother 2: ¿Tengo que comer más durante la lactancia?
[Do I have to eat more because I'm breastfeeding?]

CE: Muchas madres tienen más hambre porque están amamantando. No es necesario obligarse a comer más; simplemente coma cuando tenga hambre.
[Many mothers are more hungry because they are breastfeeding. You don't need to make yourself eat more. Just eat based on your hunger.]

CE: En sus culturas, ¿qué dice la gente acerca de los alimentos y la lactancia materna?
[In your cultures, what do people say about foods and breastfeeding?]

Mother 2: Mi mamá dice que no debería comer ni los chiles ni el puerco.
[My mom says that I shouldn't eat chili peppers or pork.]

Mother 1: Mi abuela en México me dijo que debería tomar el atole para producir más leche.
[My grandmother in Mexico said that I should drink atole in order to make more milk.]

CE: ¡O, me gusta esa bebida! Creo que es muy bueno comer los alimentos especiales para mujeres lactantes. Para mantener la producción de leche, también es importante alimentar al bebé con frecuencia.
[Oh, I like that drink! I think it's wonderful to eat special foods for nursing mothers. To keep up your supply, it's also important to feed your baby frequently.]

Mother 1: ¿Qué del alcohol y el café?
[What about alcohol and coffee?]

CE: Una bebida alcohólica de vez en cuando está bien, pero el tomar regularmente más de una puede ser peligroso para su bebé. Una taza de café al día está bien.
[An occasional alcoholic drink is okay, but regularly having more than one drink can be harmful to your baby. Having a cup of coffee a day is fine.]

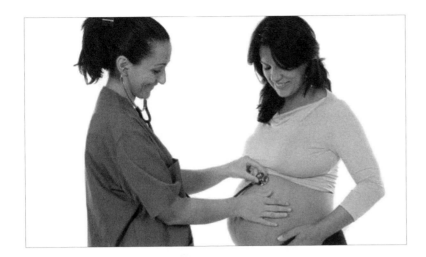

Mother 2: Mi amiga tomó un medicamento cuando estaba amamantando. ¿Eso está bien?
[My friend took a medication when she was breastfeeding. Is that okay?]

LC: Muchos medicamentos están bien, pero siempre debe consultar con su doctor acerca de los medicamentos.
[Many medications are safe, but you should always discuss medications with your doctor.]

Mother 2: ¿Qué va a pasar si no como bien? ¿Eso afecta la leche?
[What is going to happen if I don't eat well? Does that affect the milk?]

LC: Su cuerpo todavía va a producir una leche nutritiva para el bebé, pero es posible que se sienta más cansada y se enferme más. Así que trate de comer una buena dieta balanceada.
[Your body will still make nutritious milk for your baby, but you may feel more tired and get sick more often. So try to eat a good, balanced diet.]

IMPORTANT PHRASES

1. Así que .... So, therefore.

2. Puede dejar de comerlo .... You can stop eating it.

3. De vez en cuando .... Once in awhile.

4. Estaba amamantando.. She was breastfeeding.

VOCABULARY

1. afectar...to affect
2. alcohol...alcohol
3. algo.. something
4. atole ....a traditional Mexican drink
5. ayer .... yesterday
6. balanceada...............................balanced
7. bebida alcohólica ......alcoholic beverage,
8. café ....coffee
9. chile...................................chili pepper
10. cierto .... correct
11. consejos .... advice
12. consultar............................... to consult
13. cuerpo.. body
14. cultura ....culture
15. debería......................................should
16. evitar...to avoid
17. frutas...fruit
18. gases ....gas
19. gente ....people
20. granos... grains
21. medicamento......medicine, medication
22. ningún................................... no, none
23. nutritivo/a.............................nutritious
24. oír ....to hear
25. pasar .... to happen, to occur
26. peligroso............................dangerous
27. proteína...................................protein
28. puerco..pork
29. reacción .... reaction
30. regularmente ....regularly
31. salud ....health
32. se debe ....one should
33. siempre ....always
34. taza.. cup
35. tener hambre ....to be hungry
36. tener sed ....to be thirsty
37. todavía .... still, yet
38. vegetal .... vegetable

🎧 COMPREHENSION QUESTIONS

Exercise 1. After reading and listening to the dialogue on the audio file, listen again without the text and answer the following questions in Spanish. Don't worry about forming complete sentences; simply focus on writing down the key information.

Note: If you are completing the exercises in this chapter for CERPs, write your answers on the answer sheets provided in Appendix A.

1. What does the childbirth educator say about whether there are any foods in particular that breastfeeding women should avoid?

   _____

2. What kind of a diet does the childbirth educator recommend?

   _____

3. According to the childbirth educator, how much water should a breastfeeding mother drink?

   _____

4. What does the childbirth educator say about how much alcohol is safe for a breastfeeding mother to drink?

   _____

5. How does the childbirth educator respond to the question about whether a breastfeeding mother can take medications?

   _____

LANGUAGE LESSONS

A. TALKING ABOUT THE PAST: AN INTRODUCTION TO THE PAST TENSE

In Spanish, there are two ways to describe something that occurred in the past.

1. The **preterit** tense is used to describe one-time events that are now over. Often, an expression in the preterit tense will indicate a specific day or period of time in which the event took place.

2. The **imperfect** tense describes activities that used to happen or ongoing situations in the past that are now over. The imperfect tense also is used to describe personal characteristics, emotional states and age.

Study the following examples in English and see if you can distinguish the two different types of expressions in the past tense:

PRETERIT (ONE-TIME EVENTS)	IMPERFECT (ONGOING ACTIVITIES, EMOTIONAL STATES, AGE)
Yesterday, I called my doctor.	I used to live in New York.
My daughter was born last week.	I was very depressed.
I gave my son rice cereal for the first time last month.	I lived in California when I was seven.

SPANISH FOR BREASTFEEDING SUPPORT | 97

Exercise 2. Read each sentence and indicate whether it should be conjugated according to the preterit or the imperfect.

1. When I was 12, I lived in Texas.

_____

2. Last week, I had an appointment with the doctor.

_____

3. My baby was born at home.

_____

4. I was happy to breastfeed my two sons.

_____

5. I used to attend a breastfeeding support group.

_____

B. Talking about specific events in the past: The preterit tense

In this chapter, we will practice conjugating verbs in the preterit tense. In order to conjugate regular verbs in the preterit tense, we remove the ending from an unconjugated verb (*-ar, -er* or *–ir*) and add the following:

-AR VERBS		-ER/-IR VERBS	
Yo: **-é**	Nosotros: **-amos**	Yo: **-í**	Nosotros: **-imos**
Tú: **-aste**		Tú: **-iste**	
Él, Ella, Usted: **-ó**	Ellos, Ustedes: **-aron**	Él, Ella, Usted: **-ió**	Ellos, Ustedes: **-ieron**

Examples:
• El bebé **buscó** el pecho después de nacer.
[The baby looked for the breast after he was born.]

• **Pesaron** al bebé en el grupo de apoyo a la lactancia.
[They weighed the baby at the breastfeeding support group.]

• La madre **metió** el dedo en la boca del bebé para desprenderlo del pecho.
[The mother put her finger in the baby's mouth to take him off the breast.]

• **Asistí** a una clase sobre la lactancia la semana pasada.
[I attended a breastfeeding class last week.]

There are several irregular verbs and verbs with spelling changes in the preterit tense that are commonly used for breastfeeding support. Here are some examples:

IR (TO GO)		SER (TO BE)	
Yo: **fui**	Nosotros: **fuimos**	Yo: **fui**	Nosotros: **fuimos**
Tú: **fuiste**		Tú: **fuiste**	
Él, Ella, Usted: **fue**	Ellos, Ustedes: **fueron**	Él, Ella, Usted: **fue**	Ellos, Ustedes: **fueron**

Note: The conjugations of *ir* and *ser* are identical in the preterit tense. You can tell the difference between them by the context.

SACARSE (TO TAKE OUT)*		COLOCAR (TO PLACE)	
Me saqué	Nos sacamos	Coloqué	Colocamos
Te sacaste		Colocaste	
Se sacó	Se sacaron	Colocó	Colocaron

DAR (TO GIVE)		ESTAR (TO BE)	
Di	Dimos	Estuve	Estuvimos
Diste		Estuviste	
Dio	Dieron	Estuvo	Estuvieron

DECIR (TO SAY)		PRODUCIR (TO PRODUCE)	
Dije	Dijimos	Produje	Produjimos
Dijiste		Produjiste	
Dijo	Dijeron	Produjo	Produjeron

PODER (TO BE ABLE TO)		ESTAR (TO BE)	
Pude	Pudimos	Tuve	Tuvimos
Pudiste		Tuviste	
Pudo	Pudieron	Tuvo	Tuvieron

HACER (TO MAKE)		OÍR (TO HEAR)	
Hice	Hicimos	Oí	Oímos
Hiciste		Oiste	
Hizo	Hicieron	Oyó	Oyeron

* *Sacarse* is a reflexive verb. The conjugation of reflexive verbs is explained in Chapter 12. For now, it is important to focus on the spelling variations of *sacar*.

Exercise 3. Fill in the blanks with the appropriate conjugation in the preterit tense of the verb in parentheses.

1. Ayer yo _____ (llamar) al doctor.

2. Yo _____ (tener) una mancha roja en el pecho.

3. También yo _____ (sentir) escalofríos y dolores del cuerpo.

4. El doctor me _____ (dar) un antibiótico.

5. Mi hermana me _____ (decir) que tengo que descansar mucho.

6. Las madres en mi grupo de apoyo me _____ (decir) que debo tomar mucha agua.

7. El grupo de apoyo me _____ (ayudar) mucho.

8. Yo _____ (poder) dar pecho por dieciocho meses.

C. IMPERSONAL EXPRESSIONS

Impersonal expressions are a simple way to give advice in a neutral fashion. An impersonal expression says that something "is important" or "is better" instead of being a direct command.

Impersonal expressions are formed by conjugating *ser* in the third person singular (*es*) and adding an adjective, such as important, good, or bad, followed by an unconjugated verb:

Es + bueno + comer una dieta balanceada.
[It is good to eat a balanced diet.]

Examples:

• **Es importante dar pecho** a los bebés. *[It is important to breastfeed babies.]*

• **Es bueno usar** una compresa fría si tiene los pechos hinchados. *[It is good to use a cold compress if your breasts are engorged.]*

You can also put a "*no*" in front of each of these expressions to make negative statements. For example:

• **No es necesario evitar** los alimentos que causan gases. *[It is not necessary to avoid gassy foods.]*

Some common impersonal expressions are:

Es importante	It is important	Es mejor	It is better
Es necesario	It is necessary	Es bueno	It is good
Es fácil	It is easy	Es difícil	It is difficult

Exercise 4. Give some advice to a breastfeeding mother about nutrition using impersonal expressions. Write three statements by combining the expressions above (or the expressions in the negative) with one of the following endings:

• comer una dieta variada con vegetales, frutas, granos y proteína

• tomar agua cuando tiene sed

• consultar con su doctor acerca de los medicamentos

• evitar los alimentos que causan gases

Example: Es importante comer una dieta balanceada.
[It is important to eat a balanced diet.]

1. _____

2. _____

3. _____

 ## D. PRONUNCIATION PRACTICE

The Spanish language has two distinct *r* sounds—the single *r* which has a short "clip" to it, and the *rr*, which is pronounced with a trilling sound. The single *r* sound is close to a double-t sound in English. For example, the position of the tongue (the tip of the tongue touching the area behind the upper front teeth) is the same when saying "cattle" in English and *areola* in Spanish. Practice saying both words out loud to yourself and note the position of your tongue for each.

The *rr* sound requires the same positioning of the tongue, but is like a series of single *r* sounds run together and is made by repeated flaps of the tongue against the area behind the upper front teeth. Since this is an unfamiliar sound for English speakers, it may take considerable practice to produce the trilling sound.

Tongue Twisters (Trabalenguas). Listen to the following tongue twisters, making note of the different pronunciations of the single and double *r*; then repeat after the speaker, and try to keep up!

1. **Tres tristes tigres tragaban trigo en un trigal.**
   [Three sad tigers were swallowing wheat on a wheat field.]

2. **Un burro comía berros y el perro se los robó, el burro lanzó un rebuzno, y el perro al barro cayó.**
   [A donkey was eating grass and the dog stole it, the donkey brayed and the dog fell into the mud.]

LANGUAGE REVIEW: DATES

Exercise 5. Review days, months, and dates from Chapter 2. For each day and date indicated below, provide a Spanish translation.

Example: **April 3 (Tuesday):** *martes, el tres de abril*

1. November 6 (Wednesday): _____

2. October 9 (Monday): _____

3. February 1 (Thursday): _____

4. March 23 (Sunday): _____

5. July 15 (Friday): _____

 ## LISTENING COMPREHENSION

Exercise 6. Listen to the dialogue on the audio file between a mother and a childbirth educator as they discuss nutrition; then answer the comprehension questions in English.

1. What advice does the instructor have about gassy foods? _____

2. What does the mother ask about drinking water? _____

3. What does the instructor say about how much water she should drink? _____

4. What does the instructor say about drinking coffee? _____

TEAR-OUT QUICK REFERENCE: NUTRITION AND BREASTFEEDING

KEY VOCABULARY

ENGLISH	SPANISH
spicy foods	alimentos picantes
gassy foods	alimentos que causan gases
balanced diet	dieta balanceada
alcoholic drink	bebida alcohólica
coffee	café
one cup	una taza
to be hungry	tener hambre
to be thirsty	tener sed
medicine/medication	medicamento

TALKING ABOUT THE PAST: PRETERIT

-AR VERBS		-ER/-IR VERBS	
Yo: **-é**	Nosotros: **-amos**	Yo: **-í**	Nosotros: **-imos**
Tú: **-aste**		Tú: **-iste**	
Él, Ella, Usted: **-ó**	Ellos, Ustedes: **-aron**	Él, Ella, Usted: **-ió**	Ellos, Ustedes: **-ieron**

IMPERSONAL EXPRESSIONS

ES + ADJECTIVE + UNCONJUGATED VERB

It is better not to regularly drink more than one alcoholic drink while breastfeeding.	Es mejor no tomar regularmente más de una bebida alcohólica durante la lactancia.
It is not necessary to avoid certain foods while breastfeeding.	No es necesario evitar ciertos alimentos durante la lactancia.
It is important to eat a good diet with a lot of vegetables, fruits, grains, and protein.	Es importante comer una buena dieta con muchos vegetales, frutas, granos y proteína.

COMMON PHRASES

ENGLISH	SPANISH
If your baby reacts to a food, you can stop eating it for awhile.	Si su bebé tiene una reacción a un alimento, puede dejar de comerlo por un rato.
One drink once in awhile is okay, but regularly drinking more than one can be dangerous for your baby.	Una bebida alcohólica de vez en cuando está bien, pero el tomar regularmente más de una puede ser peligroso para su bebé.
You should always consult with your doctor about taking medications.	Siempre debe consultar con su doctor acerca de los medicamentos.
One cup of coffee per day is okay.	Una taza de café al día está bien.
Just drink when you are thirsty.	Simplemente tome agua cuando tenga sed.
Just eat when you are hungry.	Simplemente coma cuando tenga hambre.

NOTES FOR THE CLASSROOM INSTRUCTOR

This section is for instructors using this book in a classroom setting.

SECTION A: PRETERIT/IMPERFECT

Distinguishing between the preterit and the imperfect tense is one of the more difficult concepts for a student of Spanish to master. During this chapter, we introduce the basic concept, but only practice conjugating in the preterit tense. The next chapter explains how to conjugate the imperfect tense and provides suggestions for combining the preterit and imperfect tenses, improving the students' ability to distinguish between them and use them properly in context.

SECTION B: IMPERSONAL EXPRESSIONS

These expressions are easy to learn and involve a minimum of conjugation. There are several other impersonal expressions that can be introduced, in addition to putting "*no*" in front of them, for a wide variety of recommendations. A good exercise to do in pairs is to have one person present a problem, such as mastitis, thrush, or engorgement, and have the other student make 2-3 recommendations, using impersonal expressions.

ANSWER KEY

Need help with these exercises? Looking for more opportunities to practice? For support and additional resources to help you learn to provide breastfeeding support in Spanish, visit www.spanishforbreastfeedingsupport.com.

Exercise 1.

1. no hay ningún alimento que cause problemas a todos los bebés

2. buena, balanceada con muchas frutas, vegetales, granos y proteínas

3. cuando tiene sed

4. una bebida alcohólica de vez en cuando está bien

5. tiene que consultar con el doctor

Exercise 2.

1. Imperfect

2. Preterit

3. Preterit

4. Imperfect

5. Imperfect

Exercise 3.

1. llamé [Yesterday I called the doctor.]

2. tuve [I had a red spot on my breast.]

3. sentí [I also felt chills and body aches.]

4. dio [The doctor gave me an antibiotic.]

5. dijo [My sister said that I have to rest a lot.]

6. dijeron [The mothers in my support group told me that I should drink a lot of water.]

7. ayudó [The support group helped me a lot.]

8. pude [I was able to breastfeed for eighteen months.]

Exercise 4.

Possible starters: es importante, es necesario, es fácil, es mejor, es bueno, es difícil (each of these can also be "no es…")

Possible endings:

• comer una dieta variada con vegetales, frutas, granos, y proteína

• tomar agua cuando tiene sed

• consultar con su doctor acerca de los medicamentos

• evitar los alimentos que causan gases

Answers will vary, but some examples are:

1. Es necesario comer una dieta variada con vegetales, frutas, granos y proteína.

2. Es mejor tomar agua cuando tiene sed.

3. Es importante consultar con su doctor acerca de los medicamentos.

4. No es necesario evitar los alimentos picantes.

Exercise 5.

1. miércoles, el seis de noviembre

2. lunes, el nueve de octubre

3. jueves, el primero de febrero

4. domingo, el veintitrés de marzo

5. viernes, el quince de julio

Listening Comprehension Dialogue

Mother: Mi hermana dijo que no se debe comer alimentos que causan gases. ¿Es cierto? [My sister said that one shouldn't eat gassy foods. Is that true?]

CE: Puede comer una dieta normal. Si el bebé tiene una reacción a un alimento, puede dejar de comerlo por una rato para ver si eso ayuda. [You can eat a normal diet. If your baby has a reaction to a food, you can stop eating it for a while and see if that helps.]

Mother: Y, ¿el agua? ¿Es necesario tomar mucha agua para producir más leche? [What about water? Do you have to drink a lot of water to make more milk?]

CE: Puede tomar agua cuando tiene sed, y va a producir suficiente leche. [You can drink water when you are thirsty and you are going to make plenty of milk.]

Mother: Y, ¿el café? [And what about coffee?]

CE: Una taza de café al día está bien. [One cup of coffee a day is fine.]

Exercise 6. Answers to Comprehension Questions:

1. She can eat gassy foods. If there is a food that is causing a reaction in her baby, she can stop eating it for awhile to see if that helps.

2. She wonders whether she has to drink a lot of water.

3. The instructor says she should "drink to thirst" or when she is thirsty.

4. One cup of coffee a day is okay.

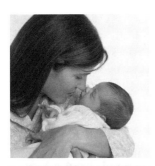

CHAPTER 9
PUMPING AND STORING BREASTMILK

By the end of
this chapter, you
will be able to:

• Understand and
use vocabulary and
phrases related
to pumping and
storing breastmilk

• Talk about ongoing
activities in the past

• Tell time and give
the time of events

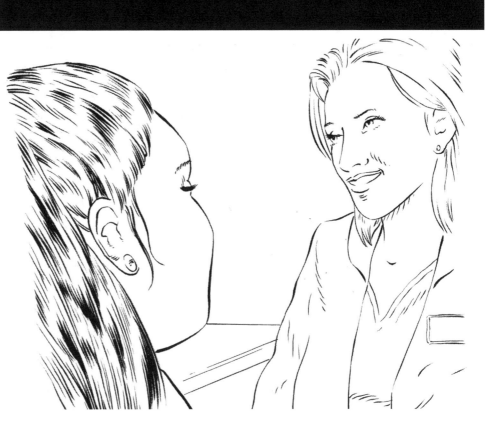

🎧 DIALOGUE

In this dialogue, a WIC Nutritionist is giving the mother of a one-month-old baby instructions on using a breastpump. Listen to the dialogue as you read along in the book. Repeat each line, pausing the audio as necessary; then listen to the vocabulary and important phrases, and repeat each one.

Setting:
• **WIC Office**

Characters:
• **WIC Nutritionist (Jean)**
• **Mother (Leticia)**
• **One-month-old baby**

WIC Nutritionist: Hola Leticia, aquí está el sacaleches alquilado para llevar a casa.
[Hi Leticia, here's the rental breastpump for you to take home.]

Mother : Gracias. ¿Me puede enseñar cómo usarlo?
[Thanks. Can you show me how to use it?]

NOTES

WIC Nutritionist: Sí. Coloque el pezón en el centro de la copa de succión. Aquí está el regulador de velocidad. Comience en una velocidad más rápida y baje la velocidad cuando vea un flujo de leche más rápido.
[Sure. Center the nipple in the flange. Here's the dial for speed. Start at a faster speed, and then slow it down when you see a faster flow of milk.]

Mother : ¿Qué hace este botón?
[What does this button do?]

WIC Nutritionist: Ese botón controla la succión. Puede ajustarlo para encontrar una presión cómoda.
[This button controls suction. You can adjust it to find a comfortable pressure.]

Mother : ¿Por cuánto tiempo debo extraer la leche?
[How long should I pump?]

WIC Nutritionist: Hasta que el flujo se reduzca bastante. Puede ser unos 10 minutos.
[Until the flow slows down a lot. That might be around 10 minutes.]

Mother : ¿Me va a doler?
[Is it going to hurt?]

WIC Nutritionist: No debe causar dolor. Si le duele, puede usar una copa de succión más grande.
[It shouldn't hurt. If it does hurt, you may need a larger flange.]

Mother : Y, ¿cómo debo de lavar las piezas?
[And how should I wash the parts?]

WIC Nutritionist: Puede lavar las piezas a mano o en el lavaplatos.
[You can wash the parts by hand or in the dishwasher.]

Mother : ¿Por cuánto tiempo puedo guardar la leche?
[How long can I keep the milk?]

WIC Nutritionist: Puede guardar la leche de cuatro a seis horas a temperatura ambiente, de tres a ocho días en el refrigerador y de seis a 12 meses en el congelador.
[You can store the milk for four to six hours at room temperature, three to eight days in the refrigerator, and six to 12 months in the freezer.]

Mother : ¿Cómo la guardo en el congelador?
[How do I store it in the freezer?]

WIC Nutritionist: Puede guardarla en bolsas de plástico para la leche materna. Como no se puede volver a congelar la leche descongelada, recomiendo congelar sólo dos o tres onzas por bolsa para no desperdiciarla.
[You can store it in breastmilk storage bags. Since you can't refreeze thawed milk, I recommend freezing only two or three ounces per bag so that you don't waste any.]

Mother : Y, ¿cómo debo calentar la leche?
[And how should I warm it up?]

WIC Nutritionist: Puede meter el biberón en un tazón de agua tibia (o "a baño María"). Pero no caliente la leche en el microondas.
[You can put the bottle in a bowl of warm water. But don't heat the milk in the microwave.]

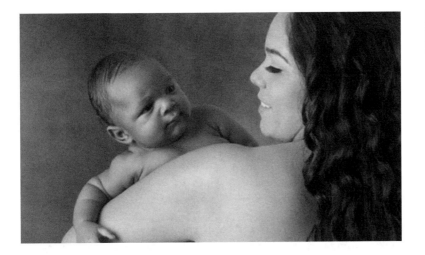

IMPORTANT PHRASES

1. Lavarlos a mano .... to wash them by hand

2. Puede usar una copa   You can use
   de succión más grande ....a larger flange.

3. Comience en una velocidad más rápida ....Start at a higher speed.

4. Baje la velocidad cuando   Lower the speed when
   vea un flujo de leche más rápido ....you see a faster flow of milk.

5. No la caliente en el microondas....... Don't heat it up in the microwave.

COMPREHENSION QUESTIONS

Exercise 1. After reading and listening to the dialogue on the audio file, listen again without the text and answer the following questions in Spanish. Don't worry about forming complete sentences; simply focus on writing down the key information.

Note: If you are completing the exercises in this chapter for CERPs, write your answers on the answer sheets provided in Appendix A.

1. What does the nutritionist say about how Leticia should set the speed of the breastpump initially?

_____

2. What does the nutritionist recommend about how long she should pump?

_____

3. What does the nutritionist suggest if it hurts to pump?

_____

VOCABULARY

1. ajustar .. to adjust (ajustarlo - to adjust it)
2. almacenamiento ....storage
3. alquilado.. rented
4. baño María......... a bowl of warm water*
5. bastante .... quite a bit, a lot
6. bolsa ....bag
7. botón...button
8. calentar................................... to heat up
9. congelador .... freezer
10. congelar .... to freeze
11. controlar ....to control
12. copa de succión ....flange
13. demasiado.............................too much
14. descongelar...........to thaw, to warm up
15. desperdiciar .... to waste
16. explicar .... to explain
17. extracción ....pumping, expression
18. flujo ....flow
19. guardar ....to keep, to store
20. lavaplatos............................ dishwasher
21. lavar........................... to wash, to clean
22. llevar.. to take
23. microondas..........................microwave
24. piezas.. parts
25. plástico ....plastic
26. presión.....................................pressure
27. rápido..fast
28. refrigerador ....refrigerator
29. regulador ....dial
30. tazón... bowl
31. temperatura ambiente.........room temperature
32. tibia ....warm
33. velocidad ....speed

Baño María is a colloquial expression that may or may not be used in your community.

4. What instructions are given about how Leticia should wash the pump parts?

_____

5. What does the nutritionist say about how Leticia can heat up the milk?

_____

LANGUAGE LESSONS

A. ONGOING ACTIVITIES IN THE PAST: THE IMPERFECT TENSE

You learned in Chapter 8 that there are two ways to describe events and occurrences in the past. The imperfect tense is used to describe what used to happen or ongoing activities in the past. It is also used to describe a person's age and physical or emotional states in the past. In order to conjugate regular verbs in the imperfect tense, we remove the ending from an unconjugated verb (-ar, -er or –ir) and add the following:

-AR VERBS		-ER/-IR VERBS	
Yo: **-aba**	Nosotros: **-ábamos**	Yo: **-ía**	Nosotros: **-íamos**
Tú: **-abas**		Tú: **-ías**	
Él, Ella, Usted: **-aba**	Ellos, Ustedes: **aban**	Él, Ella, Usted: **-ía**	Ellos, Ustedes: **-ían**

Examples:

• Yo siempre **descongelaba** la leche en un tazón de agua tibia.
[I always thawed milk in a bowl of warm water.]

• Carolina **extraía** la leche después de regresar al trabajo.
[Carolina pumped after going back to work.]

• **Vivía** en California cuando nació mi bebé.*
[I lived in California when my baby was born.]

*Note that in this sentence the imperfect tense is used in the same sentence as the preterit tense (*nació*) to denote an activity that is ongoing (living) when a single event (birth of baby) takes place.

IRREGULAR VERBS

There are only three irregular verbs in the imperfect tense, and they are commonly used.:

SER (TO BE)		VER (TO SEE)		IR (TO GO)	
Yo: **Era**	Nosotros: **Éramos**	Yo: **Veía**	Nosotros: **Veíamos**	Yo: **Iba**	Nosotros: **Íbamos**
Tú: **Eras**		Tú: **Veías**		Tú: **Ibas**	
Él, Ella, Usted: **Era**	Ellos, Ustedes: **Eran**	Él, Ella, Usted: **Veía**	Ellos, Ustedes: **Veían**	Él, Ella, Usted: **Iba**	Ellos, Ustedes: **Iban**

Exercise 2. Conjugate the verb in the imperfect tense in the following sentences.

1. Yo siempre _____ (lavar) las piezas del sacaleches en el lavaplatos.

2. Mi hermana _____ (guardar) su leche en el congelador.

3. Mi hermana y yo _____ (ir) a un grupo de apoyo a la lactancia
   hasta que nuestros bebés _____ (tener) seis meses.

4. Yo _____ (estar) triste cuando regresé al trabajo, pero el
   sacaleches me ayudó a seguir alimentando a mi bebé con leche materna.

TELLING TIME

In order to tell time in Spanish, we give the hour using the verb *ser*. For one o'clock (and all times between 1:00 and 1:59), midnight, and noon, the singular third person form of *ser* is used, while the plural is used for all other times. See the examples below:

1:00-1:59, MIDNIGHT, NOON		ALL OTHER TIMES	
Es la una.	It is one o'clock.	**Son las tres.**	It is three o'clock.
Es la medianoche.	It is midnight.	**Son las cinco.**	It is five o'clock.
Es el mediodía.	It is noon (midday).	**Son las once.**	It is eleven o'clock.

To specify morning, afternoon, and evening when giving the time, we use the following expressions:

Son las cinco **de la mañana.**	It is five in the morning.
Son las cinco **de la tarde.**	It is five in the afternoon.
Son las ocho **de la noche.**	It is eight in the evening.

In order to express that something is happening, has happened, or will happen **at** a particular time, the preposition **a** ("at") is used. Just as with telling time, the singular is used for 1:00-1:59, midnight, and noon. For example:

- Extraigo la leche a las diez, **al mediodía y a las tres.**
  [I pump at ten o'clock, noon and three o'clock.]

- Ayer, fui al doctor **a la una** de la tarde.
  [Yesterday, I went to the doctor at one in the afternoon.]

- Vamos a alimentar al bebé **a las cinco** de la mañana.
  [We are going to feed the baby at five in the morning.]

Half-hour and quarter-hour increments are expressed as follows:

Son las nueve **y media.**	It is 9:30.
Son las nueve **y cuarto.**	It is 9:15.

All other increments can be expressed with the exact number. For example:

Son las diez **y veinticinco.**	It is 10:25.
Es la una **y veinte.**	It is 1:20.
Son las doce **y cuarenta y tres.**	It is 12:43.

When telling what time it was in the past when an event occurred, the imperfect form of the verb *ser* is used. For example:

• **Eran las cuatro de la tarde** cuando llegué a casa.
[It was four in the afternoon when I got home.]

• **Era la una de la mañana** cuando el bebé se despertó.
[It was one in the morning when the baby woke up.]

Exercise 3. Write the time indicated on each clock, including what part of the day it is (morning, afternoon, evening).

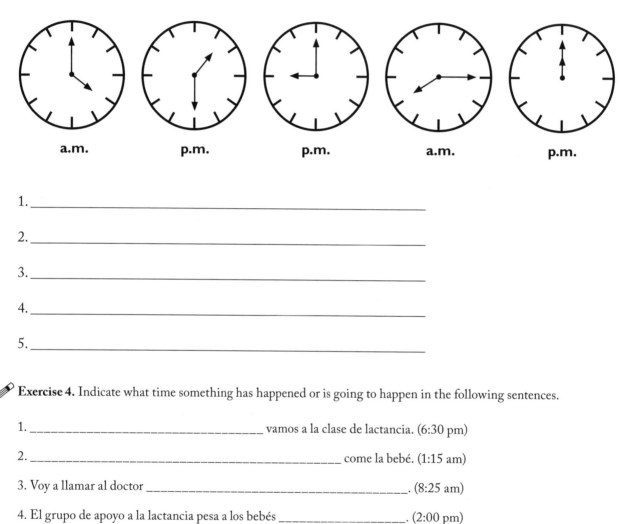

| **a.m.** | **p.m.** | **p.m.** | **a.m.** | **p.m.** |

1. _____

2. _____

3. _____

4. _____

5. _____

Exercise 4. Indicate what time something has happened or is going to happen in the following sentences.

1. _____ vamos a la clase de lactancia. (6:30 pm)

2. _____ come la bebé. (1:15 am)

3. Voy a llamar al doctor _____. (8:25 am)

4. El grupo de apoyo a la lactancia pesa a los bebés _____. (2:00 pm)

5. Anoche me saqué la leche _____. (11:00 pm)

LANGUAGE REVIEW: *TENER* EXPRESSIONS

Exercise 5. You learned about tener expressions in Chapter 6. Conjugate tener in the imperfect tense in the following sentences.

1. En marzo, mi bebé _____ (tener) cuatro meses.

2. Cuando alimenté al bebé a las tres de la mañana, _____ (tener) mucho sueño.

3. Nosotros no _____ (tener) miedo de usar el sacaleches.

4. Al principio, las madres _____ (tener) que alimentar a los bebés al menos ocho a 12 veces cada 24 horas.

5. Cuando regresé al trabajo, yo _____ (tener) que extraer la leche en la oficina.

 ## Listening Comprehension

Exercise 6. Listen to the dialogue on the audio file between a mother and a WIC nutritionist about pumping and using a breastpump; then answer the comprehension questions in English.

1. Is the mother getting a lot of milk from pumping?

   _____

2. What problem is the mother having with pumping?

   _____

3. What does the nutritionist suggest to the mother to address her problem?

   _____

4. What does the mother ask about milk storage?

   _____

5. What does the nutritionist tell her about milk storage?

   _____

Tear-Out Quick Reference: Pumping and Storing Breastmilk

KEY VOCABULARY	
ENGLISH	**SPANISH**
pumping, expression	sacarse la leche, extracción
breastpump	sacaleches
speed	velocidad
suction	succión
flow	flujo
flange	copa de succión
refrigerator	refrigerador
freezer	congelador
heat up	calentar
thaw, warm up	descongelar
warm water	agua tibia

TALKING ABOUT THE PAST: IMPERFECT			
-AR VERBS		**-ER/-IR VERBS**	
Yo: **-aba**	Nosotros: **-ábamos**	Yo: **-ía**	Nosotros: **-íamos**
Tú: **-abas**		Tú: **-ías**	
Él, Ella, Usted: **-aba**	Ellos, Ustedes: **aban**	Él, Ella, Usted: **-ía**	Ellos, Ustedes: **-ían**

TELLING TIME	
ENGLISH	**SPANISH**
It is 5:00.	Son las cinco.
It was 5:00.	Eran las cinco.
At 5:00…	A las cinco…

COMMON PHRASES	
ENGLISH	**SPANISH**
Place the nipple in the center of the flange.	Coloque el pezón en el centro de la copa de succión.
Start at a higher speed and lower the speed when you see a faster flow of milk.	Comience en una velocidad más rápida y baje la velocidad cuando vea un flujo de leche más rápido.
You can adjust the suction to find a comfortable pressure.	Puede ajustar la succión para encontrar una presión cómoda.
If it hurts, you can use a larger flange.	Si le duele, puede usar una copa de succión más grande.
Do not heat breastmilk in the microwave.	No caliente la leche materna en el microondas.
You can store the milk for 4 to 6 hours at room temperature, 3 to 8 days in the refrigerator, and 6 to 12 months in the freezer.	Puede guardar la leche de 4 a 6 horas a temperatura ambiente, de 3 a 8 días en el refrigerador y de 6 a 12 meses en el congelador.

NOTES FOR THE CLASSROOM INSTRUCTOR

This section is for instructors using this book in a classroom setting.

SECTION A: PRETERIT AND IMPERFECT TENSES: PULLING IT ALL TOGETHER

1. The preterit and imperfect tenses are taught in separate chapters in order to give students a chance to practice conjugating them in isolation. However, conceptually they must be understood together; both as forms of referring to the past.

2. A fun and instructive activity is to provide the class with a series of illustrations of a short and well-known story (for example, a fairytale). This can be put on an overhead projector or provided as a handout. Working as a class, the students will retell the story line by line, and decide whether to use the preterit or the imperfect tense for each line, generally creating one or two sentences for each illustration. The story-telling exercise demonstrates that the imperfect tense is used to describe the background scene, while the preterit tense will be used for each single action event as the story develops.

SECTION B: TELLING TIME

There are a multitude of activities that can be used in class to practice both telling time and expressing when things happen. One fun activity that gets students talking is to have each person draw a clock on a sheet of paper, with a blank line next to each of the twelve hours on the face of the clock. Next, have the students circulate around the room and make "appointments" with each other, trying to fill in each blank with the name of another student. They must conduct this conversation entirely in Spanish (e.g., "*¿Tienes una cita a las diez?*"). Once all the appointment times have been filled, the teacher calls out different times (e.g., "*¡Son las diez!*") and the students locate the person with whom they have an appointment at that time. You can assign a topic of conversation related to breastfeeding for each appointment time, such as explaining how to use a breastpump or suggestions for how to address common breastfeeding challenges.

ANSWER KEY

Need help with these exercises? Looking for more opportunities to practice? For support and additional resources to help you learn to provide breastfeeding support in Spanish, visit www.spanishforbreastfeedingsupport.com.

Exercise 1.

1. en una velocidad más rápida, reducir cuando vea un flujo más rápido

2. por 10 minutos, hasta que el flujo se reduzca bastante

3. usar una copa de succión más grande

4. en el lavaplatos o a mano

5. en un tazón de agua tibia o a baño María

Exercise 2.

1. lavaba

2. guardaba

3. íbamos

4. tenían

5. estaba

Exercise 3.

1. son las cuatro de la mañana

2. es la una y media de la tarde

3. son las nueve de la noche

4. son las ocho y cuarto de la mañana

5. es el mediodía

Exercise 4.

1. a las seis y media de la tarde

2. a la una y cuarto (or quince) de la mañana

3. a las ocho y veinticinco de la mañana

4. a las dos de la tarde

5. a las once de la noche

Exercise 5.

1. tenía

2. tenía

3. teníamos

4. tenían

5. tenía

Listening Comprehension Dialogue

WIC Nutritionist: ¿Cómo le va con la extracción de la leche?
[How is pumping going for you?]

Mother: Me va bien. Puedo extraer mucha leche.
[It's going well. I can pump a lot of milk.]

Nutritionist: ¡Excelente! Y, ¿se siente cómoda?
[That's great! And, is it comfortable for you?]

Mother: Me duele un poquito. ¿Es eso normal?
[It hurts a little bit. Is that normal?]

Nutritionist: Posiblemente necesite una copa de succión más grande. Vamos a ver (checks). Sí, creo que usted necesita una copa más grande.
[It may mean that you need a larger size flange. Let's see (checks). Yes, I think you need a larger flange.]

Mother: OK, tengo una pregunta más. ¿Por cuánto tiempo puedo guardar la leche en el refrigerador y en el congelador?
[Okay. I have one more question. How long can I keep the milk in the refrigerator and in the freezer?]

Nutritionist: Este papel explica cuánto tiempo puede guardar la leche a diferentes temperaturas.
[This sheet explains how long you can keep milk at different temperatures.]

Mother: ¡Gracias!

[Thank you!]

Exercise 6.

1. Yes, she is getting a lot of milk.

2. She is experiencing a little bit of pain when pumping.

3. The nutritionist suggests that she try a larger flange.

4. The mother wants to know how long she can store breast milk in the refrigerator and the freezer.

5. The nutritionist gives her a handout explaining how long milk can be kept at different temperatures.

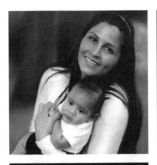

CHAPTER 10
RETURNING TO WORK

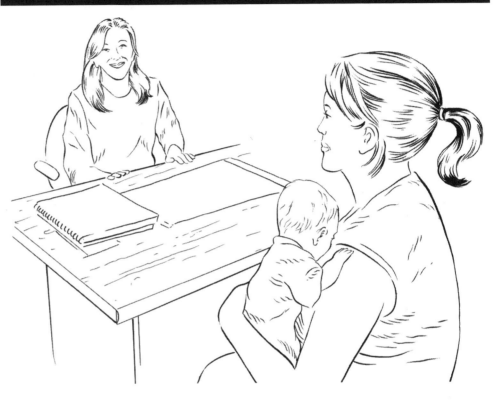

🎧 DIALOGUE

In this dialogue, a WIC breastfeeding peer counselor is helping the mother of a two-month-old baby plan to continue breastfeeding when she returns to work. Listen to the dialogue as you read along in the book. Repeat each line, pausing the audio as necessary; then listen to the vocabulary and important phrases, and repeat each one.

Setting:
• **Breastfeeding support group**

Characters:

• **WIC Breastfeeding Peer Counselor (Malia)**
• **Mother (Araceli)**
• **Two-month-old baby**

Mother: Regreso al trabajo el próximo mes y deseo platicar con usted al respecto.
[I'm going back to work next month and want to talk with you about that.]

Peer counselor: ¡Con mucho gusto le ayudo! ¿Qué ha hecho para prepararse?
[I'm happy to help! What have you done to prepare?]

Mother: Bueno, compré un doble saceleches eléctrico, y lo uso varias veces por semana. También introduje un biberón.
[Well, I bought a double electric breastpump, and I use it a few times a week. I also introduced the bottle.]

PC: ¿Su bebé se va para una guardería?
[Is your baby going to be in daycare?]

Mother: No, se va a quedar con su abuela cuando estoy en el trabajo.
[No, she's going to stay with her grandmother when I'm at work.]

PC: Excelente. ¿Cómo es su trabajo?
[Great. What is your workplace like?]

Mother: Bueno, hay una oficina que puedo usar para extraer la leche. Mi jefe me dijo que puedo extraer la leche durante los descansos y a la hora del almuerzo. ¿Cuántas veces al día debo extraer la leche?
[Well, there's an office I can use to pump. My boss said that I can pump during my breaks and at lunchtime. How many times should I pump a day?]

PC: Debe extraer la leche con la misma frecuencia que le daría de comer a la bebé en casa. En un día de trabajo, la mayoría de las madres necesitan extraer la leche tres veces.
[You should plan on pumping as often as you would be feeding the baby at home. In a full work day, most mothers need to pump three times.]

Mother: Eso va a ser difícil, pero realmente quiero hacerlo.
[That's going to be hard, but I really want to do it.]

PC: Muy bien. Así que, al final del día va a llevar la leche a casa. Ésa es la leche que la bebé va a tomar el día siguiente cuando usted está en el trabajo. Cada día extrae la leche que corresponde al próximo día.
[Great. So, at the end of the day you will bring the milk home. That's the milk she gets the next day while you are at work. Each day you pump milk for the next day.]

Mother: Ya veo.
[I see.]

PC: También puede hacer una "provisión" de leche congelada antes de regresar al trabajo, sólo por si acaso.
[You also may want to build a "back up" supply of frozen milk before you return to work, just in case.]

Mother: Yo puedo hacer eso.
[I can do that.]

PC: Cuando se acerque más la fecha de regresar al trabajo, puede dar a la bebé más práctica con el biberón.
[As you get closer to going back to work, you may want to give the baby more practice with the bottle.]

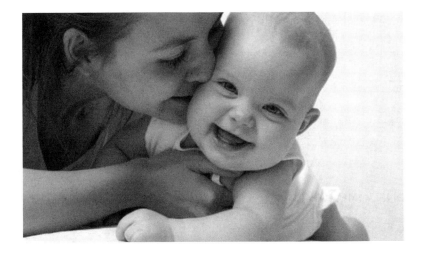

IMPORTANT PHRASES

1. El próximo mes .... next month

2. Al respecto ....about that, in that regard

3. Varias veces .... several times

4. Al final del día .... at the end of the day

5. El día siguiente.. the next day

6. Sólo por si acaso .... just in case

7. Se acerca más.. gets closer

VOCABULARY

1. abuela .... grandmother
2. almuerzo .... lunch
3. continuar .... to continue
4. descanso .... break, rest
5. difícil.......................................difficult
6. fecha.. date
7. guardería...................................daycare
8. jefe...boss
9. oficina.. office
10. platicar...........................to talk, to chat
11. práctica .... practice
12. prepararse................. to prepare oneself
13. próximo .... next
14. quedar.......................................to stay
15. querer .... to want
16. regresar................................... to return
17. regreso .... return
18. provisión.......................back up supply
19. trabajo.. work
20. vez/veces ......time, times (occurrences)

COMPREHENSION QUESTIONS

Exercise 1. After reading and listening to the dialogue on the audio file, listen again without the text and answer the following questions in Spanish. Don't worry about forming complete sentences; simply focus on writing down the key information.

Note: If you are completing the exercises in this chapter for CERPs, write your answers on the answer sheets provided in Appendix A.

1. Why is Araceli meeting with the peer counselor?

_____

2. When does Araceli plan to return to work?

_____

3. Where will her baby stay while she is at work?

_____

4. What does the peer counselor say about how many times most mothers need to pump at work each day?

_____

5. What are some additional things that Araceli can do in preparation?

_____

LANGUAGE LESSONS

A. EXPRESSING THAT YOU HAVE DONE SOMETHING

We use the present perfect tense to express having done something. For example:

- I have rented a breastpump.
- Marta has returned to work.

There are two steps required to form the present perfect tense.

First, we conjugate *haber*, or "to have," according to the person who has taken the action or done the activity. Here is the present tense conjugation of *haber*:

HABER	
Yo: **He**	Nosotros: **Hemos**
Tú: **Has**	
Él, Ella, Usted: **Ha**	Ellos, Ustedes: **Han**

Note: The verb *haber* is used as "to have" when talking about having done something, while *tener* expresses "to have" an object.

Second, we form the past participle of the action word (in the examples above, "rented" and "returned"). To form the past participle of regular verbs, remove the ending of an unconjugated verb and attach *–ado* to *–ar* verbs and *–ido* to *–er* and *–ir* verbs.

Examples:

-AR VERBS		-ER/-IR VERBS	
Hablar	Hablado	Comer	Comido
Alimentar	Alimentado	Dormir	Dormido
Alquilar	Alquilado	Producir	Producido

IRREGULAR VERBS AND SPELLING CHANGES IN THE PAST PARTICIPLE FORM

There are a few irregular verbs in the past participle form that are commonly used for breastfeeding support:

IRREGULAR PAST PARTICIPLES	
VERB	PAST PARTICIPLE
Hacer	Hecho
Poner	Puesto
Ver	Visto
Abrir	Abierto
Decir	Dicho

In addition, there are three verbs that require an accent in the past participle form:

Verb	Past Participle
Oir	Oído
Traer	Traído
Creer	Creído

Examples:

  • **Hemos oído** que hay ciertos alimentos que no debemos comer durante la lactancia.
  [*We have heard that there are certain foods we should not eat while breastfeeding.*]

  • La doctora me **ha dicho** que puedo seguir amamantando después de regresar al trabajo.
  [*The doctor has told me that I can keep breastfeeding after going back to work.*]

Exercise 2. Conjugate the verb in the present perfect tense in the following sentences.

Example:

  • Nosotras _____ (regresar) al trabajo.

  • Nosotras *hemos regresado* al trabajo.

1. Ana _____ (amamantar) por seis meses.

2. Mi mama me _____ (decir) que es mejor evitar los alimentos que causan gases durante la lactancia.

3. Yo _____ (alquilar) un sacaleches para llevar al trabajo.

4. Los bebés _____ (aumentar) de peso cada semana.

5. Nosotras _____ (oír) que se puede tomar algunos medicamentos durante la lactancia, pero que es mejor consultar con su doctor.

B. This and These: Demonstrative Adjectives

The words "this" (*este, esta*) and "these" (*estos, estas*) are used to describe people or things that are close to the speaker or in his or her possession. These adjectives agree in number and gender with the object or person being described. Here are some examples:

  • **Este** sacaleches es fácil de usar.
  [*This breastpump is easy to use.*]

  • **Estas** piezas se pueden lavar a mano o en el lavaplatos.
  [*These parts can be washed by hand or in the dishwasher.*]

  • **Este** doctor le va a ayudar.
  [*This doctor is going to help you.*]

Exercise 3. Fill in the blanks with the appropriate form of "this" or "these" in Spanish.

1. _____ antibiótico le va a ayudar con la infección.

2. Para controlar la presión, use _____ botón.

3. _____ enfermera me ayudó a dar pecho.

4. _____ madres tienen preguntas acerca del almacenamiento de la leche.

5. _____ pañales están sucios.

C. That and Those: Demonstrative Adjectives

The words "that" (*ese, esa*) and "those" (*esos, esas*) are used to describe people or things that are at a slight distance. These adjectives also agree in number and gender with the object or person being described. Here are some examples:

> • **Esos** reguladores en el sacaleches son para velocidad y succión.
> [*Those dials on the breastpump are for speed and suction.*]

> • **Esa** consultora de lactancia es muy buena.
> [*That lactation consultant is very good.*]

Exercise 4. Fill in the blanks with the appropriate form of "that" or "those" in Spanish.

1. Lleve _____ sacaleches al trabajo para extraer la leche durante los descansos.

2. _____ bebés comen ocho veces por día.

3. Use _____ compresa fría para el hinchazón.

4. _____ mancha roja en el pecho es síntoma de una infección.

5. _____ copas de succión son muy grandes para usted.

Language Review: Formal Commands

Exercise 5. You learned how to give formal commands in Chapter 3. Conjugate the verbs as singular formal commands in the following sentences to guide a mother in using a breastpump.

1. _____ (usar) este sacaleches en el trabajo.

2. _____ (poner) el pezón en el centro de la copa de succión.

3. _____ (comenzar) en una velocidad más rápida.

4. _____ (controlar) la presión con este botón.

5. _____ (lavar) las piezas del sacaleches a mano o en el lavaplatos.

Listening Comprehension

Exercise 6. Listen to the dialogue on the audio file between a mother and a breastfeeding peer counselor as they discuss going back to work; then answer the comprehension questions in English.

1. What has the mother done to prepare for returning to work?

   _____

2. Where will the mother be pumping?

   _____

3. Where will the baby stay when the mother goes back to work?

   _____

4. What did the mother's boss tell her about time she can take to pump?

   _____

5. What did the peer counselor tell the mother about the number of times she will need to pump?

   _____

Tear-Out Quick Reference: Returning to Work

KEY VOCABULARY	
ENGLISH	**SPANISH**
work, job	trabajo
office	oficina
break	descanso
lunch	almuerzo
boss	jefe
daycare	guardería
bottle	biberón

Talking About What Someone Has Done: Present Perfect

HABER			PAST PARTICIPLE	
Yo: **He**	Nosotros: **Hemos**		Regular **-ar**	**-ado**
Tú: **Has**			Regular **-er and -ir**	**-ido**
Él, Ella, Usted: **Ha**	Ellos, Ustedes: **Han**			

COMMON IRREGULAR PAST PARTICIPLE FORMS			
Hacer	Hecho	Poner	Puesto
Decir	Dicho	Ver	Visto
Abrir	Abierto		

This/That/These/Those: Demonstrative Adjectives

This: **Este/Esta**	These: **Estos/Estas**
That: **Ese/Esa**	Those: **Esos/Esas**

Common Phrases

ENGLISH	SPANISH
What have you done to prepare yourself?	¿Qué ha hecho para prepararse?
What is your workplace like?	¿Cómo es su trabajo?
You should pump with the same frequency as you would feed the baby at home.	Debe extraer la leche con la misma frecuencia que le daría de comer a la bebé en casa.
In a full work day, most mothers need to pump three times.	En un día de trabajo, la mayoría de las madres necesitan sacarse la leche tres veces.
At the end of the day, you will bring the milk home. That's the milk she will get the next day.	Al final del día va a llevar la leche a casa. Ésa es la leche que va a tomar el día siguiente.
You also can build a "back up" supply of frozen milk before you return to work.	También puede hacer un provisión de leche congelada antes de regresar al trabajo.
As you get closer to going back to work, you may want to give the baby more practice with the bottle.	Cuando se acerque más la fecha de regresar al trabajo, puede dar a la bebé más práctica con el biberón.

Notes for the Classroom Instructor

This section is for instructors using this book in a classroom setting.

Section A: Present Perfect Tense

1. As part of your classroom warm-up exercises, you can ask students to tell something about themselves in the present perfect tense (for example, something exceptional they may have done during their lives).

2. Another way to help students learn the present perfect tense in context is to have them read excerpts from articles or stories that include it. Ask them to note the ways in which the present perfect tense is used. One good source of clear and easy-to-read Spanish is *Selecciones* by Reader's Digest. This magazine contains short articles from the medical field that use some of the important vocabulary taught in the breastfeeding context, as well as providing well-written articles that can be used in many ways in the classroom.

3. In general, a good way to help students improve their reading comprehension and develop spoken fluency is to ask them to read a short piece and "re-tell" it to you in Spanish—essentially, they will summarize the story. These will not be perfect recitations, but you can focus on different grammatical structures each time you repeat the exercise.

ANSWER KEY

Need help with these exercises? Looking for more opportunities to practice? For support and additional resources to help you learn to provide breastfeeding support in Spanish, visit www.spanishforbreastfeedingsupport.com.

Exercise 1.

1. va a regresar al trabajo

2. el próximo mes

3. con su abuela

4. tres veces

5. dar a la bebé más práctica con el biberón; hacer una provisión de leche

Exercise 2.

1. ha amamantado

2. ha dicho

3. he alquilado

4. han aumentado

5. hemos oído

Exercise 3.

1. Este

2. Este

3. Esta

4. Estas

5. Estos

Exercise 4.

1. ese

2. Esos

3. esa

4. Esa

5. Esas

Exercise 5.

1. Use

2. Ponga

3. Comience

4. Controle

5. Lave

Listening Comprehension Dialogue

Peer counselor: ¿Cómo se ha preparado para regresar al trabajo?
[How have you prepared for going back to work?]

Mother: Estoy usando un sacaleches y he introducido un biberón.
[I am pumping and have introduced a bottle.]

Peer counselor: ¡Muy bien! ¿Puede extraer la leche en el trabajo?
[Great! Can you pump at work?]

Mother: Sí, puedo sacarme la leche en mi oficina.
[Yes, I can pump in my office.]

Peer counselor: ¿Dónde se va a quedar la bebé mientras está en el trabajo?
[Where will the baby stay while you are at work?]

Mother: Se va para una guardería.
[She is going to daycare.]

Peer counselor: ¿Ha platicado con su jefe acerca de la extracción de la leche?
[Have you talked with your boss about pumping?]

Mother: Sí, dice que puedo usar mis descansos y la hora del almuerzo. ¿Es suficiente si me saco la leche tres veces en el trabajo?
[Yes, he says that I can use my breaks and lunch time. Is it enough to pump three times at work?]

Peer counselor: Sí, normalmente tres veces es suficiente.
[Yes. Normally, three times is enough.]

Exercise 6.

1. She has started pumping and has introduced a bottle.

2. In her office at work

3. The baby will go to daycare.

4. He said she could use her break times and lunch time to pump.

5. Three times during the day is usually enough.

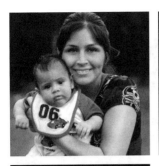

CHAPTER 11
STARTING COMPLEMENTARY FOODS

By the end of this chapter, you will be able to:

• Understand and use vocabulary and phrases related to starting complementary foods

• Express likes and dislikes

• Use the conditional tense to express "should"

• Recognize common prepositions

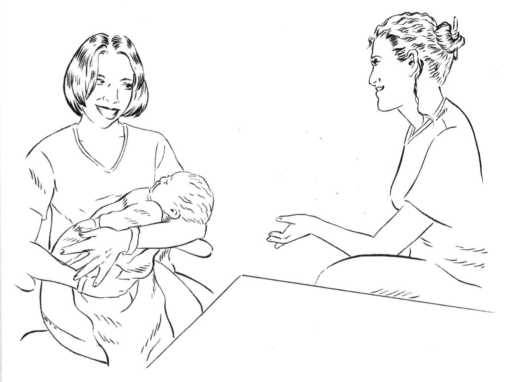

🎧 DIALOGUE

In this dialogue, the mother of a six-month-old baby is asking a lactation counselor some questions about introducing solid foods at a breastfeeding support group meeting. Listen to the dialogue as you read along in the book. Repeat each line, pausing the audio as necessary; then listen to the vocabulary and important phrases, and repeat each one.

Setting:
• **Breastfeeding support group**

Characters:

• **Lactation counselor (Anita)**
• **Mother (Nina)**
• **Five-month-old baby**

Mother: Me gustaría hablar de cuándo introducir los alimentos sólidos. Me parece que mi bebé podría estar listo pronto.
[*I'd like to talk about when to start solid foods. It seems like my baby could be ready soon.*]

Counselor: Sí. La mayoría de los bebés están listos para comenzar los alimentos sólidos a los seis meses aproximadamente.
[*Sure. Most babies are ready to start solids at around six months.*]

NOTES

Mother: ¿Cómo puedo saber cuándo está listo?
[How do I know when he's ready?]

Counselor: Cuando los bebés están listos, normalmente demuestran un interés en la comida, pueden sentarse y no escupen la comida.
[When babies are ready, they usually show interest in food, are able to sit up, and don't spit out the food.]

Mother: O, tiene mucho interés en nuestra comida. Me mira cuando estoy comiendo todo el tiempo y trata de agarrar mi comida.
[Oh, he's really interested in our food. He watches me eat all the time and grabs at my food.]

Counselor: Muy bien.
[That's great.]

Mother: ¿Cuándo debo ofrecerle alimentos sólidos?
[When should I offer him some solid food?]

Counselor: Trate de darle alimentos sólidos entre las comidas de pecho. Deje que juegue con la comida y se divierta.
[Try giving him solids in between breastfeedings. Let him play with the food and have fun.]

Mother: ¿Qué le debería dar primero?
[What should I give him first?]

Counselor: Puede comenzar con una fruta o vegetal machacado como camote, plátano o aguacate en forma de puré, o un cereal. Puede mezclar la leche materna con estos alimentos también.
[You can start with a pureed fruit or vegetable, like sweet potato, banana, or avocado, or a cereal. You can also mix breastmilk into these foods.]

Mother: Y, ¿cuánto debería darle?
[And how much should I give him?]

Counselor: Al principio, sólo una cucharadita* al día está bien, y puede aumentar la cantidad de ahí. Recomiendo introducir las comidas una por una por unos días para ver si su bebé tiene una reacción.
[At first, just a teaspoon a day is fine, and you can increase the amount from there. I recommend introducing the foods one at a time for a few days, so you can see if your baby has a reaction to it.]

Mother: ¿Qué hago si no quiere comer los alimentos sólidos?
[What do I do if he doesn't want to eat the solid food?]

Counselor: Está bien. Deje que el bebé explore y juegue con la comida, y no le obligue a comer.
[That's okay. Let him play with it and explore, and don't force him to eat.]

** Other recommendations include a tablespoon (*una cucharada*) and "as much as he wants," (*la cantidad que quiera el bebé.)*

IMPORTANT PHRASES

1. Todo el tiempo .... all the time

2. Al principio .... at first

3. Uno por uno (or una por una).. one at a time

4. Por unos días ....for a few days

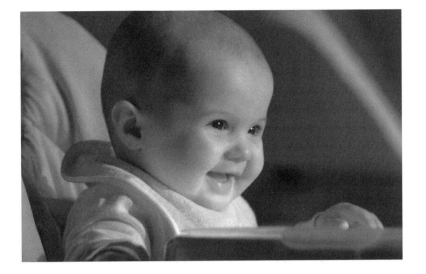

COMPREHENSION QUESTIONS

Exercise 1. After reading and listening to the dialogue on the audio file, listen again without the text and answer the following questions in Spanish. Don't worry about forming complete sentences; simply focus on writing down the key information.

Note: If you are completing the exercises in this chapter for CERPs, write your answers on the answer sheets provided in Appendix A.

1. When does the lactation counselor say that most babies are ready for solid foods?

_____

2. What cues does the lactation counselor tell Nina to look for in order to tell if her baby is ready for solid foods?

_____

3. What advice does the lactation counselor give about how to introduce solid foods?

_____

4. What does the lactation counselor say about how much solid food Nina should give her baby at first?

_____

5. What advice does the lactation counselor give to Nina about what to do if her baby doesn't want to eat solid foods?

_____

VOCABULARY

1. agarrar...to grab

2. aguacate.....................................avocado

3. camote...............................sweet potato

4. cereal..cereal

5 comida de pecho,   feeding
   toma, lactada ....(breastfeeding)

6. cualquier...any

7. cucharadita ....teaspoon

8. demostrar ....to demonstrate

9. divertirse ....to have fun

10. escupir ....to spit out

11. explorar................................ to explore

12. fruta...fruit

13. gustar............................. to be pleasing

14. interés .... interest

15. jugar ....to play

16. mezclar.......................................to mix

17. obligar.. to obligate, to force, to require

18. plátano.....................................banana

19. poder...................................to be able to

20. puré de,   mashed,
   en forma de puré .... pureed

21. querer.. to want

22. sentarse......................... to sit, to sit up

LANGUAGE LESSONS

A. EXPRESSING LIKES AND DISLIKES

The verb *gustar* in Spanish is used to express likes and dislikes. However, instead of saying that a person "likes something," we say that something "is pleasing to" that person. In other words, it is the object that is liked that performs the action of being pleasing.

For example, in order to say, "I like vegetables," you would write: *Me gustan los vegetales*. The literal translation of this sentence is "Vegetables please me." That is why the verb *gustar* is conjugated in the plural form (*gustan*). The *me* refers to the person who is pleased, in this case, "me."

Here are the words to place in front of *gustar* to indicate who is pleased:

Yo: **me**	Nosotros: **nos**
Tú: **te**	
Él, Ella, Usted: **le**	Ellos, Ustedes: **les**

When expressing likes or dislikes of objects in the present tense, the verb *gustar* is conjugated as either *gusta* for singular or *gustan* for more than one object.

Examples:

> • **Le gusta** el sacaleches eléctrico.
> [*She likes the electric breastpump.*]

> • **No les gusta** el café.
> [*They do not like coffee.*]

In order to express liking or disliking an action (verb), the singular form of *gustar* (*gusta*) is used, as in the following examples:

> • **Me gusta alimentar** al bebé cuando llego del trabajo.
> [*I like to feed my baby when I get home from work.*]

> • **Nos gusta probar** nuevos alimentos.
> [*We like to try new foods.*]

You'll notice that when using *le* or *les* in front of gustar, it's not entirely clear who is doing the liking. *Le* could refer to he, she, or the formal "you" (*usted*), while *les* could refer to they (masculine or feminine) or the plural "you all." In order to identify the person doing the liking, we can add *a + the person doing the liking*, as in the following examples:

> • **A la bebé** le gusta comer frutas en forma de puré.
> [*The baby likes to eat pureed fruit.*]

> • **A muchos bebés** les gustan los cereales.
> [*Many babies like cereals.*]

You can also add the person simply for extra emphasis:

> • **A mi** no me gusta el cereal.
> [*I don't like cereal.*]

Exercise 2. Estela is a breastfeeding mother who is reporting her likes and dislikes of certain foods to you. Conjugate the verb *gustar* with *me* in the following sentences. Example: *Me gusta la leche.*

1. _____ los vegetales.

2. También _____ algunas frutas.

3. No _____ la banana (banana).

4. _____ la zanahoria (carrot).

5. _____ mucho las manzanas y peras (apples and pears).

Exercise 3. Fill in the blanks in the following paragraph to describe the food preferences of a group of women in a breastfeeding support group.

A Clara _____ las frutas y los vegetales. Ella dice que sus favoritos son las manzanas y los aguacates.

A Clara no _____ la carne, pero sí _____ comer el pescado, a veces. A las otras mujeres

_____ la carne (beef), el pollo (chicken) y los mariscos (seafood). A todas nosotras _____

preparar la comida en casa.

B. Another way to give recommendations and advice

The conditional tense expresses "would" or "could," and also can be used to express "should," when used with the verb *deber*. The conjugation of the conditional tense is very simple; just add the following endings to the unconjugated form of the verb:

Yo: **ía**	Nosotros: **íamos**
Tú: **ías**	
Él, Ella, Usted: **ía**	Ellos, Ustedes: **ían**

A good way to give polite recommendations is with *deber*.

Examples:

- Las madres **deberían** esperar hasta los seis meses, aproximadamente, antes de introducir alimentos complementarios.
[*Mothers should wait until about six months before introducing complementary foods.*]

- **Debería** seguir amamantando a demanda.
[*You should continue to breastfeed on cue.*]

- No **deberíamos** obligar a los bebés a comer alimentos sólidos.
[*We shouldn't force babies to eat solid foods.*]

Exercise 4. Fill in the blanks with the correct conjugation of the verb *deber* to find out what the following people should do.

1. Nosotras _____ introducir los alimentos sólidos cuando el bebé demuestra un interés en la comida, puede sentarse y no escupe la comida.

2. Los bebés no _____ necesitar más que la leche materna por los primeros seis meses.

3. Yo _____ introducir los alimentos uno por uno al principio.

4. Marisa no _____ obligar a su bebé a comer alimentos sólidos.

5. El bebé _____ poder sentarse antes de introducir los alimentos sólidos.

C. Prepositions

Prepositions are connector words that generally describe the relationship of one object to another in time (before, after) or in space (over, under). You already have been exposed to many prepositions in the various dialogues presented in this book. Typically, prepositions are the last thing that a student masters in another language; therefore, we are providing only a brief list to guide you. The following are some of the most common prepositions:

en	at, in
de	from, of, about
con	with
sin	without
a, al*	to, at, per
por	for, per, about, by
para	for, in order to
entre	between
sobre	over
bajo	under
después de	after
antes de	before
durante	during
hasta	until

*A note about *a* and *al*: *al* is used when the word following *a* is masculine (*el*). The *a* combines with *el* to form *al*. Example: *Voy [a + el] al hospital.*

Examples:

- Voy **al** hospital.
[*I'm going **to** the hospital.*]

- El bebé está **en** brazos de su mamá.
[*The baby is **in** his mother's arms.*]

- Los bebés necesitan comer ocho a 12 veces **por** día.
[*Babies need to eat eight to 12 times **per** day.*]

LANGUAGE REVIEW: PAST TENSE (PRETERIT) AND TELLING TIME

Exercise 5. Using the preterit tense that you learned in Chapter 8 and time expressions from Chapter 9, write a sentence indicating what a breastfeeding mother who is working outside the home did at each of the following times.

Example: 8:30 am (trabajo): A las ocho y media de la mañana, fue al trabajo.

1. 7:00 am (amamantar a su bebé): _____

2. 12:00 pm (usar el sacaleches): _____

3. 5:30 pm (regresar a casa): _____

4. 6:30 pm (comer): _____

5. 9:30 pm (descansar): _____

LISTENING COMPREHENSION

Exercise 6. Listen to the dialogue on the audio file between a mother and a lactation counselor as they discuss starting complementary foods; then answer the comprehension questions in English.

1. How old is the baby?

_____

2. What does the mother want to know?

_____

3. What does the lactation counselor say about breastmilk?

_____

4. What does the lactation counselor say about the baby's readiness for solids?

_____

5. What does the mother conclude about the baby's readiness for solids?

_____

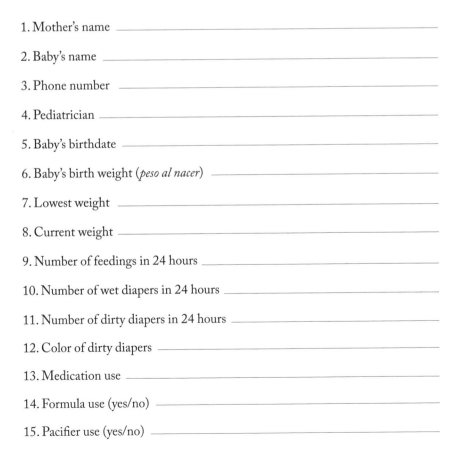 **Exercise 7.** Breastfeeding Intake Exercise

In this exercise, you will listen to a conversation between a mother and a breastfeeding support person. The support person is gathering information about the mother and baby to complete an intake form. Listen to their conversation. Fill in the answers on the intake form in English.

Breastfeeding Intake Form

1. Mother's name _____

2. Baby's name _____

3. Phone number _____

4. Pediatrician _____

5. Baby's birthdate _____

6. Baby's birth weight (*peso al nacer*) _____

7. Lowest weight _____

8. Current weight _____

9. Number of feedings in 24 hours _____

10. Number of wet diapers in 24 hours _____

11. Number of dirty diapers in 24 hours _____

12. Color of dirty diapers _____

13. Medication use _____

14. Formula use (yes/no) _____

15. Pacifier use (yes/no) _____

Tear-Out Quick Reference: Starting Complementary Foods

KEY VOCABULARY	
ENGLISH	**SPANISH**
solid foods	alimentos sólidos
to introduce	introducir
pureed fruits	frutas en forma de puré
pureed vegetables	puré de vegetales
teaspoon	cucharadita
tablespoon	cucharada
reaction	reacción

LIKES AND DISLIKES: GUSTAR	
Yo: **me gusta/me gustan**	Nosotros: **nos gusta/nos gustan**
Tú: **te gusta/te gustan**	
Él, Ella, Usted: **le gusta/le gustan**	Ellos, Ustedes: **les gusta/les gustan**

ANOTHER WAY TO EXPRESS SHOULD: CONDITIONAL	
Yo: **debería**	Nosotros: **deberíamos**
Tú: **deberías**	
Él, Ella, Usted: **debería**	Ellos, Ustedes: **deberían**

COMMON PREPOSITIONS			
a, al	Voy **al** hospital.	**en**	El bebé está **en** brazos de su mamá.
con	Ponga al bebé piel **con** piel.	**de**	El sacaleches es **de** Sara.
hasta	Los bebés aumentan una onza por día **hasta** los tres meses.	**por**	Es mejor introducir los alimentos uno **por** uno.

COMMON PHRASES	
ENGLISH	**SPANISH**
Most babies are ready to start solid foods at around six months.	La mayoría de los bebés están listos para comenzar los alimentos sólidos a los seis meses aproximadamente.
When babies are ready, they show interest in food, are able to sit up, and don't spit out the food.	Cuando los bebés están listos, demuestran un interés en la comida, pueden sentarse y no escupen la comida.
Breastmilk gives him all the nutrition he needs for the first six months.	La leche materna le da toda la nutrición que necesita por los primeros seis meses.
You can start with a pureed fruit or vegetable, or a cereal.	Puede comenzar con una fruta o vegetal en forma de puré o un cereal.
At first, just a tablespoon a day is fine, and then increase from there.	Al principio, sólo una cucharada al día está bien, y puede aumentar la cantidad de ahí.
Let him explore and play with it, and don't force him to eat.	Deje que el bebé explore y juegue con la comida, y no le obligue a comer.

NOTES FOR THE CLASSROOM INSTRUCTOR

This section is for instructors using this book in a classroom setting.

SECTION A: *GUSTAR*

Discussing likes and dislikes is well-suited for a classroom activity in pairs. Students can ask each other about various activities, foods, books, and movies they like. They can also discuss whether they like common first foods, such as bananas, cereal, fruits, and vegetables, to practice the vocabulary in Spanish.

SECTION B: CONDITIONAL TENSE

One exercise for the classroom that will allow students to practice *deber* in the conditional tense in a breastfeeding context is to pose some of the "breastfeeding challenges" from Chapter 7 and ask the students to discuss how mothers should address the challenge. Some examples of challenges include engorgement, sore or cracked nipples, and symptoms of mastitis.

SECTION C: PREPOSITIONS

1. One activity for teaching prepositions is to take an object and place it in different places in relation to a table or desk; then ask the students where it is, i.e., "over" or "under" the table/desk.

2. In addition, students can listen to the dialogues from previous chapters in class and have a contest to see who can pick out the most prepositions. Research in second language acquisition suggests that prepositions should be learned by seeing and using the words in context. For that reason, we provide only a brief discussion with some of the more common prepositions used for breastfeeding support.

ANSWER KEY

Need help with these exercises? Looking for more opportunities to practice? For support and additional resources to help you learn to provide breastfeeding support in Spanish, visit www.spanishforbreastfeedingsupport.com.

Exercise 1.

1. a los seis meses

2. demuestra interés en la comida, puede sentarse, no escupe la comida

3. uno por uno, entre las comidas de pecho, fruta o vegetal en forma de puré primero

4. una cucharadita al día

5. no le obligue; dejar que explore y juegue

Exercise 2.

1. Me gustan

2. me gustan

3. me gusta

4. Me gusta

5. Me gustan

Exercise 3.

1. le gustan

2. le gusta

3. le gusta

4. les gustan

5. nos gusta

Exercise 4.

1. deberíamos

2. deberían

3. debería

4. debería

5. debería

Exercise 5.

1. A las siete de la mañana amamantó a su bebé.

2. Al mediodía, usó el sacaleches.

3. A las cinco y media de la tarde, regresó a casa.

4. A las seis y media de la tarde, comió.

5. A las nueve y media de la noche, descansó.

Listening Comprehension Dialogue

Mother: ¿Está listo mi bebé para los alimentos sólidos? Tiene tres meses.
[Is my baby ready for solid foods? He's three months old.]

Lactation counselor: Normalmente, los bebés están listos cuando tienen seis meses.
[Usually babies are ready when they are six months old.]

Mother: ¿Es suficiente la leche materna?
[Is breastmilk enough?]

Lactation counselor: Sí. Recibe toda la nutrición que necesita de su leche.
[Yes. He gets all the nutrition he needs from your milk.]

Mother: ¿Cómo puedo saber cuándo está listo?
[How can I know when he's ready?]

Lactation counselor: Cuando tiene interés en su comida, puede sentarse, y no escupe la comida.
[When he shows interest in your food, can sit up, and doesn't spit out food.]

Mother: Creo que él no está listo todavía.
[I think he's not ready yet.]

Exercise 6.

1. The baby is three months old.

2. She wants to know whether her baby is ready for solid foods.

3. Breastmilk provides all the nutrition the baby needs at this stage.

4. The baby will be ready for solids when he shows an interest in food, can sit up, and does not spit food out.

5. He's not ready yet.

Breastfeeding Intake Dialogue

Q: Hola. ¿Cómo se llama?
A: Me llamo Lupita Díaz.

Q: ¿Cómo se llama su bebé?
A: Se llama Laura Díaz.

Q: ¿Cuál es su número de teléfono?
A: Es el (723) 845-9933.

Q: ¿Cómo se llama el doctor de su bebé?
A: Se llama el Dr. Cantú.

Q: ¿Cuándo nació su bebé?
A: El seis de octubre.

Q: ¿Cuánto pesó la bebé al nacer?
A: Pesó ocho libras con tres onzas.

Q: ¿Cuánto fue el peso más bajo de la bebé?
A: Creo que siete libras con siete onzas.

Q: ¿Cuánto pesa su bebé ahora?
A: Ahora pesa ocho libras con nueve onzas.

Q: ¿Cuántas veces alimenta a la bebé en 24 horas?
A: 7 veces.

Q: ¿Cuántos pañales mojados hace la bebé en 24 horas?
A: Más o menos 10.

Q: ¿Cuántos pañales sucios hace la bebé en 24 horas?
A: Creo que 7.

Q: ¿De qué color son los pañales sucios de la bebé?
A: Son de un color amarillo-anaranjado.

Q: ¿Está tomando usted o su bebé algún medicamento?
A: Yo estoy tomando una vitamina; mi bebé no toma nada.

Q: ¿La bebé toma fórmula?
A: No.

Q: ¿La bebé usa un chupón?
A: Sí, pero no mucho.

Exercise 7.

1. Mother's name: Lupita Díaz

2. Baby's name: Laura Díaz

3. Phone number: (723) 845-9933

4. Pediatrician: Dr. Cantú

5. Baby's birthdate: October 6

6. Baby's birth weight (peso al nacer): 8 lbs., 3 ozs.

7. Lowest weight: 7 lbs., 7 ozs.

8. Current weight: 8 lbs., 9 ozs.

9. Number of feedings in 24 hours: 7 times

10. Number of wet diapers in 24 hours: 10, more or less

11. Number of dirty diapers in 24 hours: 7

12. Color of dirty diapers: yellow-orange

13. Medication use: Mother: Vitamin, Baby: nothing

14. Formula use (yes/no): No

15. Pacifier use (yes/no): Yes, but not much

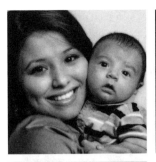

CHAPTER 12
WEANING

OBJECTIVES

By the end of this chapter, you will be able to:

• Understand and use vocabulary and phrases related to weaning

• Talk about the future and future plans

• Recognize and use reflexive verbs

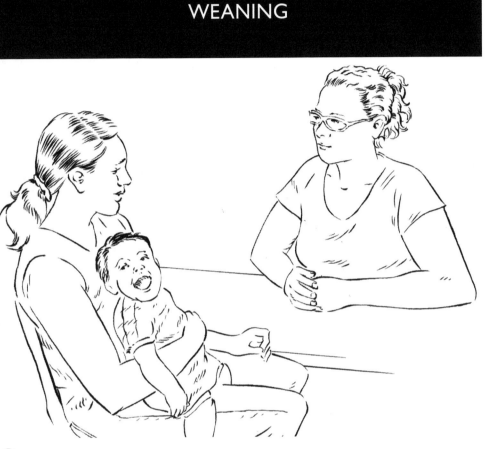

🎧 DIALOGUE

In this dialogue, the mother of an 18-month-old baby discusses weaning with a breastfeeding support group leader. Listen to the dialogue as you read along in the book. Repeat each line, pausing the audio as necessary; then listen to the vocabulary and important phrases, and repeat each one.

Setting:
• **Breastfeeding support group**

Characters:

• **Group Leader (Megan)**
• **Mother (Dulce)**
• **Five-month-old baby**

Leader: Hola, Dulce. ¿Cómo le va con la lactancia?
[Hi Dulce. How is breastfeeding going for you?]

Mother: Me ha ido muy bien, pero creo que estoy lista para destetar al bebé.
[It's been great, but I think I'm ready to wean now.]

Leader: Me alegra que la lactancia le haya ido bien. Tengo algunas sugerencias acerca de cómo destetar al bebé. ¿Con qué frecuencia lo está amamantando ahora?
[I'm happy to hear that breastfeeding has gone well for you. I have some suggestions for you about how to wean. How often is he nursing now?]

Mother: El bebé amamanta un par de veces por día, principalmente en la noche y en la mañana.
[He's nursing a couple of times a day, mostly at night and in the morning.]

Leader: Es importante destetar al bebé poco a poco. Así, los pechos y el bebé se acostumbrarán al cambio.
[It's important to wean the baby gradually. That way, both the baby and your breasts will adjust to the change.]

Mother: ¿Qué significa "poco a poco"?
[What do you mean by "gradually"?]

Leader: Puede quitarle una toma cada dos o tres días. Trate de distraerlo a las horas en que normalmente le daría pecho y déle muchos cariños.
[You can cut out one nursing every 2 or 3 days. Try distracting him at nursing times, and give him lots of love.]

Mother: OK. Creo que podré hacer eso, pero será más difícil de noche.
[Okay. I think I'll be able to do that, but it'll be harder at night.]

Leader: Tal vez podría comenzar con la toma de la mañana
[Maybe you could start with the morning feeding.]

Mother: ¿Qué debería hacer si los pechos se sienten muy llenos?
[What should I do if I feel full?]

Leader: Si se sienten muy llenos, puede usar el sacaleches o extraer un poco de leche a mano para aliviar la presión.
[If you ever feel very full, you can pump or hand express a little to relieve the pressure.]

Mother: ¿Eso mantendrá la producción de leche?
[Will that keep my supply going?]

Leader: No afectará mucho la producción, y ayudará a evitar los conductos obstruídos y la mastitis.
[It won't affect your supply very much, and it will help prevent plugged ducts and mastitis.]

IMPORTANT PHRASES

1. Me ha ido muy bien..................................It has gone very well for me.

2. Un par de veces por día ....a couple of times a day

3. Cada dos o tres días...every few days

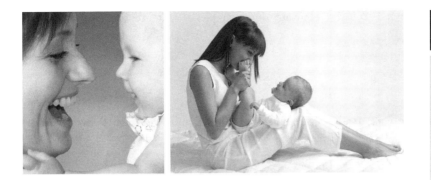

COMPREHENSION QUESTIONS

Exercise 1. After reading and listening to the dialogue on the audio file, listen again without the text and answer the following questions in Spanish. Don't worry about forming complete sentences; simply focus on writing down the key information.

Note: If you are completing the exercises in this chapter for CERPs, write your answers on the answer sheets provided in Appendix A.

1. How is breastfeeding going for Dulce?

_____

2. How often is Dulce's baby breastfeeding right now?

_____

3. What does the support group leader say about how Dulce should go about weaning her baby?

_____

4. What advice is given about which feeding Dulce should eliminate first?

_____

5. What does the support group leader say that Dulce should do if her breasts feel full?

_____

LANGUAGE LESSONS

A. ANOTHER WAY TO TALK ABOUT THE FUTURE

In Chapter 7, you learned how to use *ir+a* to express what you are going to do. There is also a future tense that can be used to express future plans. The future tense of regular verbs is formed by taking an unconjugated verb and adding the following endings:

Yo: **é**	Nosotros: **emos**
Tú: **ás**	
Él, Ella, Usted: **á**	Ellos, Ustedes: **án**

VOCABULARY

1. acostumbrarse ... to get used to, to adjust
2. aliviar .... to relieve
3. cariños .... affection
4. destetar.................................... to wean
5. destete .... weaning
6. distraer .... to distract
7. eliminar .... to eliminate
8. juntos.. together
9. lleno.. full
10. mantener .... to maintain
11. poco a poco..... gradually, little by little
12. principalmente .... mostly, mainly
13. sugerencia........................... suggestion
14. tiempo .... time

These endings are used with regular *-ar, -er* and *-ir* verbs. Here are some examples of sentences in the future tense:

- Silvia **destetará** al bebé poco a poco.
[*Silvia will wean the baby gradually.*]

- Ella también **introducirá** alimentos sólidos.
[*She also will introduce solid foods.*]

The list below contains six stem-changing verbs in the future tense that are the most common in breastfeeding support. The future tense endings are added to the stems of these verbs as modified:

decir (to say)	dir-
hacer (to make, to do)	har-
poder (to be able to)	podr-
saber (to know a fact)	sabr-
poner (to put, to place)	pondr-
tener (to have)*	tendr-

* Like *tener*, the words *mantener* (to maintain), *contener* (to contain) and *obtener* (to obtain) are also stem-changing in the future and conditional tenses and have similar stems (*mantendr-, contendr-, obtendr-*).

Examples:

- Fabiola **podrá** sacarse la leche en el trabajo.
[*Fabiola will be able to pump at work.*]

- Ella **pondrá** el sacaleches en su oficina.
[*She will put the breastpump in her office.*]

Exercise 2. Conjugate the verbs in the future tense in the following sentences.

1. Si el destete se hace poco a poco, el bebé se _____ (acostumbrar) al cambio.

2. Si los pechos se sienten llenos, la extracción manual de la leche _____ (aliviar) la presión.

3. Para comenzar el destete, nosotras _____ (eliminar) una comida de pecho cada dos o tres días.

4. A veces los pechos se _____ (sentir) muy llenos durante el proceso del destete.

5. Yo _____ (tener) que distraer al bebé a las horas de comer.

B. REFLEXIVE VERBS

Certain verbs require a special conjugation called the reflexive. Some are verbs in which the person performing an action is also the recipient of the action, as in "to bathe oneself" or "to take care of oneself." In addition, there are certain expressions that always require a reflexive construction, such as describing how someone feels (*sentirse*) or saying someone's name (*llamarse*).

When conjugating a reflexive verb, you must take the *se*, which is attached to the end of the unconjugated form, place it in front of the verb, and make it agree with the person who is the recipient of the action. These words are called reflexive pronouns.

REFLEXIVE PRONOUNS	
Yo: **me**	Nosotros: **nos**
Tú: **te**	
Él, Ella, Usted: **se**	Ellos, Ustedes: **se**

The reflexive pronouns in self-care verbs are substitutes for "myself," "yourself," "herself," "himself," "ourselves" and "themselves."

Examples:

- *Se cuida bien*. [*She takes care of herself.*]
- *Nos bañamos*. [*We take a bathe (we bathe ourselves).*]
- *Me siento* triste. [*I feel sad.*]

There are several common reflexive verbs in the breastfeeding context:

COMMON REFLEXIVE VERBS	
acostarse	to lay down
acostumbrarse	to accustom oneself, to get used to
bañarse	to bathe oneself
cuidarse	to take care of oneself
levantarse	to get up
limpiarse	to wash oneself
llamarse	to call oneself, to be named
preocuparse	to feel worried
sacarse	to take out, to pump milk
sentarse	to sit down
sentirse	to feel an emotion

Examples:

- **Me levanto** a las ocho de la mañana.
  [*I get up at eight in the morning.*]

- Carla **se siente** lista para destetar a su bebé.
  [*Carla feels ready to wean her baby.*]

- A veces las madres **se preocupan** por sus bebés durante el destete.
  [*Sometimes, mothers worry about their babies during weaning.*]

Exercise 3. Conjugate the reflexive verbs in the present tense in the following sentences.

1. Gabriela _____ (sentirse) un poco triste.

2. Yo estoy lista para destetar a mi bebé, pero también _____ (preocuparse).

3. La líder del grupo de apoyo a la lactancia dice que los bebés _____ (acostumbrarse) mejor al destete cuando es poco a poco.

4. Nosotras _____ (levantarse) a las seis de la mañana.

5. Lilia _____ (bañarse) a las seis y media, así que va a eliminar la toma de la mañana.

LANGUAGE REVIEW: PRETERIT AND IMPERFECT TENSES

Exercise 4. You'll recall from Chapter 9 that the imperfect tense is used to describe repetitive activities, age, and emotional states in the past, while the preterit tense describes specific actions or events that take place. In other words, the imperfect tense is the backdrop, while the preterit tense is the action taking place on that backdrop. In the following narrative, conjugate the verbs in parentheses in either the preterit or imperfect tense.

1. Yo _____ (ir) a un grupo de apoyo a la lactancia cada lunes.

2. En cada reunión, nosotras _____ (hablar) de los retos y éxitos (successes) con la lactancia.

3. Cuando mi bebé _____ (tener) dieciocho meses, yo estaba lista para el destete.

4. Para comenzar, yo _____ (eliminar) la toma de la mañana.

5. Mi bebé _____ (acostumbrarse) rápidamente al cambio.

🎧 LISTENING COMPREHENSION

Exercise 5. Listen to the dialogue on the audio file between a mother and a breastfeeding support group leader as they discuss weaning; then answer the comprehension questions in English.

1. What does the mother want to do?

_____

2. How does the leader suggest she do it?

_____

3. What does the leader mean by "gradually"?

_____

4. What does the leader suggest the mother do as she reduces feedings?

_____

5. What is the mother's final question?

_____

Exercise 6. Breastfeeding Intake Exercise

In this exercise, you will listen to a conversation between a mother and a breastfeeding support person. The support person is gathering information about the mother and baby to complete an intake form. Listen to their conversation. Fill in the answers on the intake form in English.

Breastfeeding Intake Form

1. Mother's name _____
2. Baby's name _____
3. Phone number _____
4. Pediatrician _____
5. Baby's birthdate _____
6. Baby's birth weight (*peso al nacer*) _____
7. Lowest weight _____
8. Current weight _____
9. Number of feedings in 24 hours _____
10. Number of wet diapers in 24 hours _____
11. Number of dirty diapers in 24 hours _____
12. Color of dirty diapers _____
13. Medication use _____
14. Formula use (yes/no) _____
15. Amount _____
16. Pacifier use (yes/no) _____

Tear-Out Quick Reference: Weaning

KEY VOCABULARY	
ENGLISH	**SPANISH**
weaning	destete
to wean	destetar
feeding	comida de pecho, toma
to eliminate	quitar, eliminar
to distract	distraer
full	lleno
gradually, little-by-little	poco a poco

FUTURE TENSE ENDINGS	
Yo: **-é**	Nosotros: **-emos**
Tú: **-ás**	
Él, Ella, Usted: **-á**	Ellos, Ustedes: **-án**

REFLEXIVE PRONOUNS	
Yo: **me**	Nosotros: **nos**
Tú: **te**	
Él, Ella, Usted: **se**	Ellos, Ustedes: **se**

COMMON REFLEXIVE VERBS	
bañarse (to bathe oneself)	acostumbrarse (to become accustomed)
levantarse (to get up)	sentirse (to feel an emotion)
sentarse (to sit oneself down)	preocuparse (to feel worried)
cuidarse (to take care of oneself)	sacarse (to pump milk)

COMMON PHRASES	
ENGLISH	**SPANISH**
How often is he nursing now?	¿Con qué frecuencia está amamantando ahora?
It's important to wean the baby gradually.	Es importante destetar al bebé poco a poco.
You can cut out one nursing every few days.	Puede quitarle una toma cada dos o tres días.
If your breasts feel very full, you can pump or hand express to relieve the pressure.	Si los pechos se sienten muy llenos, puede usar el sacaleches o extraer la leche a mano para aliviar la presión.

Notes for the Classroom Instructor

This section is for instructors using this book in a classroom setting.

Section A: Future Tense

A fun classroom exercise with the future tense is to ask the students to write a short sentence or two explaining what they will do tomorrow, next week, next month, next year, or in five or ten years. They can pick something general or specific, but it must be in the future tense. Then working in pairs, the students will interview each other and find out the future plans of their partner. Finally, each student will make a brief presentation to describe the future plans of their partner to the class. This allows the students to practice the future tense in the first person, second person, and third person, as well as use question words.

Section B. Reflexive Verbs

This chapter focuses on the proper use of reflexive pronouns, while keeping the verb itself in the present tense. Classroom exercises can expand upon this by having the students conjugate the verbs in other tenses.

1. Ask the students to write a brief schedule, indicating what they did at different times during the day. They can also describe what they will do tomorrow, thereby bringing in the future tense. This is especially good for the "self-care" verbs (getting up, bathing, etc.) that tend to be reflexive.

2. A common warm-up exercise for the beginning of each class is to ask students, *¿Cómo te sientes?* Make sure to point out to the students that this is a reflexive construction. If you have not been using it to warm up the class each day, it is a good exercise to practice expressing emotions and conditions.

ANSWER KEY

Need help with these exercises? Looking for more opportunities to practice? For support and additional resources to help you learn to provide breastfeeding support in Spanish, visit www.spanishforbreastfeedingsupport.com.

Exercise 1.

1. bien, está lista para destetar al bebé

2. un par de veces por día

3. poco a poco

4. de la mañana

5. usar el sacaleches o extraer la leche a mano

Exercise 2.

1. acostumbrará

2. aliviará

3. eliminaremos

4. sentirán

5. tendré

Exercise 3.

1. se siente

2. me preocupo

3. se acostumbran

4. nos levantamos

5. se baña

Exercise 4.

1. iba

2. hablábamos

3. tenía

4. eliminé

5. se acostumbró

Listening Comprehension Dialogue

Mother: Creo que estoy lista para destetar al bebé. ¿Cómo debo hacerlo?
[I think I'm ready to wean the baby. How should I do it?]

Leader: Recomiendo destetar al bebé poco a poco.
[I recommend weaning the baby gradually.]

Mother: ¿Por qué?
[Why?]

Leader: Ayudará a su bebé y a los pechos a acostumbrarse.
[It will help your baby and your breasts adjust.]

Mother: OK. ¿Cómo debería hacerlo?
[Okay. How should I do it?]

Leader: Puede eliminar una comida de pecho cada dos o tres días.
[You can cut out one feeding every few days.]

Mother: ¿Debo distraerlo a las horas de comer?
[Should I distract him at feeding times?]

Leader: Sí, es una buena idea. Y asegúrese de darle más cariños.
[Yes, that's a good idea. And be sure to give him more affection.]

Mother: ¿Qué hago si los pechos se sienten muy llenos?
[What do I do if my breasts feel full?]

Leader: Puede extraer la leche con un sacaleches o a mano para aliviar la presión.
[You can pump or hand express to relieve the pressure.]

Exercise 5.

1. The mother wants to wean her baby.

2. The leader suggests that the mother wean gradually.

3. Cutting one feeding every few days.

4. She should distract him at meal times and give the baby lots of affection.

5. What should she do if she feels full?

Breastfeeding Intake Dialogue

Q: Hola. ¿Cómo se llama?
A: Me llamo Nina Santos.

Q: ¿Cómo se llama su bebé?
A: Se llama Pablo Santos.

Q: ¿Cuál es su número de teléfono?
A: Es el (703) 332-5567.

Q: ¿Cómo se llama el doctor de su bebé?
A: Se llama la doctora Birney.

Q: ¿Cuándo nació su bebé?
A: El quince de febrero.

Q: ¿Cuánto pesó el bebé al nacer?
A: Pesó seis libras con tres onzas.

Q: ¿Cuánto fue el peso más bajo del bebé?
A: Creo que cinco libras con diez onzas.

Q: ¿Cuánto pesa su bebé ahora?
A: Ahora pesa siete libras con dos onzas.

Q: ¿Cuántas veces alimenta al bebé en 24 horas?
A: Más o menos 12 veces.

Q: ¿Cuántos pañales mojados hace el bebé en 24 horas?
A: Aproximadamente 10.

Q: ¿Cuántos pañales sucios hace el bebé en 24 horas?
A: Creo que 6 o 7.

Q: ¿De qué color son los pañales sucios del bebé?
A: Son de un color amarillo-anaranjado.

Q: ¿Está tomando usted o su bebé algún medicamento?
A: No, no tomamos ningún medicamento.

Q: ¿El bebé toma fórmula?
A: Sí.

Q: ¿Cuánta fórmula?
A: Le doy más o menos seis onzas por día.

Q: ¿El bebé usa un chupón?
A: Sí, a veces.

Exercise 6.

1. Mother's name: Nina Santos

2. Baby's name: Pablo Santos

3. Phone number: (703) 332-5567

4. Pediatrician: Dr. Birney

5. Baby's birthdate: February 15

6. Baby's birth weight (peso al nacer): 6 lbs., 3 ozs.

7. Lowest weight: 5 lbs., 10 ozs.

8. Current weight: 7 lbs., 2 ozs.

9. Number of feedings in 24 hours: 12

10. Number of wet diapers in 24 hours: about 10

11. Number of dirty diapers in 24 hours: 6-7

12. Color of dirty diapers: yellow-orange

13. Medication use: No

14. Formula use (yes/no): Yes

15. Amount: 6 ozs./day

16. Pacifier use (yes/no): Yes, sometimes

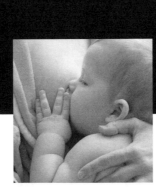

REFERENCES FOR THE INTRODUCTION

Centers for Disease Control and Prevention, National Immunization Survey, Breastfeeding among children born 1999-2005.

Feldman-Winter, L. (2004, November). Breastfeeding Care in the Delivery Hospital Environment. Presented at the annual meeting of the American Public Health Association.

Galvin, S., Grossman, X., Feldman-Winter, L., Chaudhuri, J., & Merewood, A. (2008). A practical intervention to increase breastfeeding initiation among Cambodian women in the U.S. *Maternal and Child Health Journal, 12:4*, 545-547.

Krashen, S. D. (2004, November). *Applying the Comprehension Hypothesis: Some Suggestions.* 13th International Symposium and Book Fair on Language Teaching (English Teachers Association of the Republic of China), Taipei, Taiwan.

Spartley, E., Johnson, A., Sochalski, J., Fritz, M., Spencer, W. (2000). The Registered Nurse Population. Washington, D.C.: U.S. Department of Health and Human Services.

U.S. Census Bureau. (2004). Census Bureau projects tripling of Asian and Hispanic populations in 50 years, non-Hispanic whites may drop to half of total population. Washington, D.C.: U.S. Census Bureau

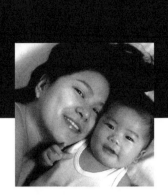

APPENDICES

APPENDIX A
CERPs for International Board Certified Lactation Consultants

Each chapter of this book meets the criteria for L-CERPs and has been approved as an independent study module. International Board Certified Lactation Consultants may earn CERPs for completing these modules. CERP forms are provided in this section of the book and on the website: www.spanishforbreastfeedingsupport.com. You can either tear out or copy the forms in this section or download the forms from the website.

This book been approved for 12.8 L-CERPs by Hale Publishing, a long-term provider approved by the International Board of Lactation Consultant Examiners. Each chapter offers approximately 1 L-CERP and will take you approximately 1 hour to complete. The number of L-CERPs earned for the completion of each chapter (0.9 – 1.3) is listed on the Self-Directed Evaluation for each chapter.

To earn CERPs for completing some or all of the chapters in this book, fill out the following CERP forms:

1. self-assessment questionnaire form (submit only one, even if submitting several chapters)

2. answer sheet for each chapter

3. self-directed evaluation for each chapter

Instructions:

1. Jot down the time you start and end each chapter module, including time to read through the chapter and complete the exercises.

    Time started chapter module: _____

    Time finished chapter module:_____

    Time to complete chapter module: _____

Put this information on the evaluation sheet.

2. Read the chapter.

3. On the Answer Sheet for the chapter, enter your answers to the exercises in the chapter.

4. Check your answers using the Answer Key at the end of each chapter. If you miss any answers, reread that section in the chapter and retake that portion of the exercise. You must answer 70% correctly to get continuing education credit for the chapter module.

5. Complete the Self Assessment Questionnaire and the Self-Directed Evaluation.

6. For each chapter module you complete, send your completed Self-Assessment Questionnaire Form (only one if sending multiple chapters at one time), Answer Sheet (one for each chapter), Self-Directed Evaluation (one for each chapter), and check for $20.00 (per chapter) or credit card information to:

Hale Publishing
1712 N. Forest St.
Amarillo, TX 79106

7. You will be sent a Certificate of Successful Completion for each chapter you complete. Please keep the certificates on file.

SELF-ASSESSMENT QUESTIONNAIRE FORM
SPANISH FOR BREASTFEEDING SUPPORT
HALE PUBLISHING

Name: _____

Credentials: _____ Date of birth: _____

Address: _____

City: _____ State:____ Postal Code: _____

Country: _____ Phone: _____

Email: _____

Lactation Consultant - year certified:_____

Are you currently employed in a setting related to lactation? __ Yes __ No

How many years have you worked with breastfeeding families? ___

What is the highest educational level you have achieved?

__ High School Diploma __ Undergraduate Degree __ Master's Degree __ Doctorate Degree

To receive L-CERPs, please submit the following:

1. This form (if submitting for multiple chapters at the same time, complete form only once)

2. Answer sheet for each chapter completed

3. Self-directed evaluation for each chapter completed

4. Payment (see below)

The cost to receive continuing education credit for each chapter is $20.

Number of chapters completed: ____   Number of CERPs requested: ___

Method of Payment:

___ Check   Check number: _____

___ Credit Card: ___ Visa ___ Master Card

Credit Card Number: _____

Expiration date: _____ Authorized signature: _____

Return this form, answer sheet(s), evaluation form(s), and check (if paying by check) to:

Hale Publishing
1712 Forest Street
Amarillo, TX 79106

CHAPTER 1 ANSWER SHEET
SPANISH FOR BREASTFEEDING SUPPORT

Name:

Need help with these exercises? Looking for more opportunities to practice? Visit www.spanishforbreastfeedingsupport.com for support and additional resources to help you learn to provide breastfeeding support in Spanish.

EXERCISE 1

1. a. b. c. d.

2. _____

3. a. b. c. d.

EXERCISE 2

1. ___ ___ ___ ___

2. ___ ___ ___ ___ ___

3. ___ ___ ___ ___ ___ ___

4. ___ ___ ___ ___ ___ ___

5. ___ ___ ___ ___ ___

EXERCISE 3

1. _____ areola

2. _____ cabeza

3. _____ pezón

4. _____ labios

5. _____ enfermeras

EXERCISE 4

1. _____ madre

2. _____ pecho

3. _____ lengua

4. _____ alvéolos

5. _____ doctoras

EXERCISE 5

Glossary Term	Gender (m or f)	"The"
1. Pezón		_____ pezón
2. Nariz		_____ nariz
3. Mano		_____ mano
4. Calostro		_____ calostro
5. Problema		_____ problema
6. Familia		_____ familia
7. Alergia		_____ alergia
8. Pañal		_____ pañal
9. Padre		_____ padre
10. Piel		_____ piel

CHAPTER 1 ANSWER SHEET, PAGE 2
SPANISH FOR BREASTFEEDING SUPPORT

EXERCISE 6

1. _____ 6. _____ 11. _____

2. _____ 7. _____ 12. _____

3. _____ 8. _____ 13. _____

4. _____ 9. _____ 14. _____

5. _____ 10. _____ 15. _____

EXERCISE 7

1. _____

2. _____

3. _____

4. _____

5. _____

CHAPTER 1 SELF-DIRECTED EVALUATION
SPANISH FOR BREASTFEEDING SUPPORT

TITLE: CHAPTER 1

L-CERPs: 0.9

Location:

Date:

Purpose of the activity: To help breastfeeding support professionals effectively support breastfeeding mothers in Spanish.

Please complete this evaluation questionnaire. Your anonymous responses will be used to revise this activity and to plan for future educational activities. Circle the number that best fits your evaluation of this activity.

1 Not at all   2 Somewhat   3 Almost completely   4 Completely

1. Rate your achievement of these objectives:				
a. Understand and use vocabulary and phrases related to the baby and the breast	1	2	3	4
b. Pronounce the sounds of the Spanish alphabet	1	2	3	4
c. Talk about people and things	1	2	3	4
d. Count from one to 31	1	2	3	4
2. Rate the effectiveness of teaching/learning resources.	1	2	3	4
3. Were the objectives relevant to the overall purpose?	1	2	3	4
4. Was the material new to you?	1	2	3	4
5. Will you be able to use this information in your work setting?	1	2	3	4

6. How many independent study modules have you completed? _____

7. Are you interested in completing more independent study modules? __ yes ___ no

8. How long did it take you to complete this module? _____ hours _____ minutes

9. Comments on the module. If you answered 1 to any of the above, please comment below:

CHAPTER 2 ANSWER SHEET
SPANISH FOR BREASTFEEDING SUPPORT

Name:

Need help with these exercises? Looking for more opportunities to practice? Visit www.spanishforbreastfeedingsupport.com for support and additional resources to help you learn to provide breastfeeding support in Spanish.

EXERCISE 1

1. a. b. c. d.

2. a. b. c. d.

3. a. b. c. d.

4. a. b. c. d.

5. a. b. c. d.

EXERCISE 2

1. _____

2. _____

3. _____

4. _____

5. _____

6. _____

7. _____

EXERCISE 3

1. _____

2. _____

3. _____

4. _____

5. _____

EXERCISE 4

1. _____

2. _____

3. _____

4. _____

5. _____

EXERCISE 5

1. _____

2. _____

3. _____

4. _____

5. _____

CHAPTER 2 ANSWER SHEET, PAGE 2
SPANISH FOR BREASTFEEDING SUPPORT

EXERCISE 6

1. _____
2. _____
3. _____
4. _____
5. _____

EXERCISE 7

1. _____
2. _____
3. _____
4. _____
5. _____

EXERCISE 8

1. a. b. c. d.
2. a. b. c. d.
3. a. b. c. d.
4. a. b. c. d.

EXERCISE 9

1. a. b. c. d.
2. a. b. c. d.
3. a. b. c. d.

SELF-DIRECTED EVALUATION
SPANISH FOR BREASTFEEDING SUPPORT

TITLE: CHAPTER 2

L-CERPs: 1.3

Location:

Date:

Purpose of the activity: To help breastfeeding support professionals effectively support breastfeeding mothers in Spanish.

Please complete this evaluation questionnaire. Your anonymous responses will be used to revise this activity and to plan for future educational activities. Circle the number that best fits your evaluation of this activity.

1 Not at all   2 Somewhat   3 Almost completely   4 Completely

1. Rate your achievement of these objectives:				
a. Understand and use vocabulary and phrases related to positioning	1	2	3	4
b. Refer to people and things	1	2	3	4
c. Use basic action words	1	2	3	4
d. Understand and use days of the week and months of the year	1	2	3	4
2. Rate the effectiveness of teaching/learning resources.	1	2	3	4
3. Were the objectives relevant to the overall purpose?	1	2	3	4
4. Was the material new to you?	1	2	3	4
5. Will you be able to use this information in your work setting?	1	2	3	4

6. How many independent study modules have you completed? _____

7. Are you interested in completing more ISMs? __ yes ___ no

8. How long did it take you to complete this module? _____ hours _____ minutes

9. Comments on the module. If you answered 1 to any of the above, please comment:

CHAPTER 3 ANSWER SHEET
Spanish for Breastfeeding Support

Name:

Need help with these exercises? Looking for more opportunities to practice? Visit www.spanishforbreastfeedingsupport.com for support and additional resources to help you learn to provide breastfeeding support in Spanish.

EXERCISE 1

1. a. b. c. d.

2. a. b. c. d.

3. a. b. c. d.

4. a. b. c. d.

5. a. b. c. d.

EXERCISE 2

1. _____

2. _____

3. _____

4. _____

5. _____

EXERCISE 3

1. _____

2. _____

3. _____

4. _____

5. _____

6. _____

7. _____

EXERCISE 4

1. _____   6. _____

2. _____   7. _____

3. _____   8. _____

4. _____   9. _____

5. _____   10. _____

EXERCISE 5

1. _____

2. _____

3. _____

4. _____

5. _____

CHAPTER 3 ANSWER SHEET, PAGE 2
SPANISH FOR BREASTFEEDING SUPPORT

EXERCISE 6

1. _____

2. _____

3. _____

4. _____

EXERCISE 7

Breastfeeding Intake Form

1. Mother's name _____

2. Baby's name _____

3. Phone number _____

4. Pediatrician _____

5. Baby's birthdate _____

SELF-DIRECTED EVALUATION
SPANISH FOR BREASTFEEDING SUPPORT

TITLE: CHAPTER 3

L-CERPs: 1.1

Location:

Date:

Purpose of the activity: To help breastfeeding support professionals effectively support breastfeeding mothers in Spanish.

Please complete this evaluation questionnaire. Your anonymous responses will be used to revise this activity and to plan for future educational activities. Circle the number that best fits your evaluation of this activity.

1 Not at all   2 Somewhat   3 Almost completely   4 Completely

1. Rate your achievement of these objectives:				
a. Understand and use vocabulary and phrases related to latch	1	2	3	4
b. Give basic commands	1	2	3	4
c. Count from 31 to 100	1	2	3	4
d. Recognize colors	1	2	3	4
2. Rate the effectiveness of teaching/learning resources.	1	2	3	4
3. Were the objectives relevant to the overall purpose?	1	2	3	4
4. Was the material new to you?	1	2	3	4
5. Will you be able to use this information in your work setting?	1	2	3	4

6. How many independent study modules have you completed? _____

7. Are you interested in completing more ISMs?   ___ yes ___ no

8. How long did it take you to complete this module? _____ hours _____ minutes

9. Comments on the module. If you answered 1 to any of the above, please comment:

CHAPTER 4 ANSWER SHEET
SPANISH FOR BREASTFEEDING SUPPORT

Name:

Need help with these exercises? Looking for more opportunities to practice? Visit www.spanishforbreastfeedingsupport.com for support and additional resources to help you learn to provide breastfeeding support in Spanish.

EXERCISE 1

1. _____
2. _____
3. _____
4. _____
5. _____

EXERCISE 2

1. _____
2. _____
3. _____
4. _____
5. _____
6. _____

EXERCISE 3

1. _____
2. _____
3. _____
4. _____
5. _____
6. _____

EXERCISE 4

1. _____
2. _____
3. _____
4. _____
5. _____

EXERCISE 5

1. _____
2. _____
3. _____
4. _____
5. _____

CHAPTER 4 ANSWER SHEET, PAGE 2
SPANISH FOR BREASTFEEDING SUPPORT

EXERCISE 6

1. _____

2. _____

3. _____

4. _____

EXERCISE 7

1. _____

2. _____

3. _____

4. _____

5. _____

EXERCISE 8

Breastfeeding Intake Form

1. Mother's name _____

2. Baby's name _____

3. Phone number _____

4. Pediatrician _____

5. Baby's birthdate _____

6. Baby's birth weight _____

7. Number of feedings in 24 hours _____

8. Formula use (yes/no) _____

9. Amount _____

SELF-DIRECTED EVALUATION
SPANISH FOR BREASTFEEDING SUPPORT

TITLE: CHAPTER 4

L-CERPs: 1.1

Location:

Date:

Purpose of the activity: To help breastfeeding support professionals effectively support breastfeeding mothers in Spanish.

Please complete this evaluation questionnaire. Your anonymous responses will be used to revise this activity and to plan for future educational activities. Circle the number that best fits your evaluation of this activity.

1 Not at all   2 Somewhat   3 Almost completely   4 Completely

1. Rate your achievement of these objectives:				
a. Understand and use vocabulary and phrases related to feeding frequency and duration	1	2	3	4
b. Describe people and things	1	2	3	4
c. Use *ser* and *estar* and understand the difference	1	2	3	4
d. Use question words	1	2	3	4
2. Rate the effectiveness of teaching/learning resources.	1	2	3	4
3. Were the objectives relevant to the overall purpose?	1	2	3	4
4. Was the material new to you?	1	2	3	4
5. Will you be able to use this information in your work setting?	1	2	3	4

6. How many independent study modules have you completed? _____

7. Are you interested in completing more ISMs? __ yes ___ no

8. How long did it take you to complete this module? _____ hours _____ minutes

9. Comments on the module. If you answered 1 to any of the above, please comment:

CHAPTER 5 ANSWER SHEET
Spanish for Breastfeeding Support

Name:

Need help with these exercises? Looking for more opportunities to practice? Visit www.spanishforbreastfeedingsupport.com for support and additional resources to help you learn to provide breastfeeding support in Spanish.

EXERCISE 1

1. _____
2. _____
3. _____
4. _____
5. _____

EXERCISE 2

1. _____
2. _____
3. _____
4. _____
5. _____

EXERCISE 3

1. _____
2. _____
3. _____
4. _____
5. _____

EXERCISE 4

1. _____
2. _____
3. _____
4. _____
5. _____

EXERCISE 5

1. _____
2. _____
3. _____
4. _____
5. _____

CHAPTER 5 ANSWER SHEET, PAGE 2
SPANISH FOR BREASTFEEDING SUPPORT

EXERCISE 6

1. _____

2. _____

3. _____

4. _____

5. _____

EXERCISE 7

1. _____

2. _____

3. _____

4. _____

EXERCISE 8

Breastfeeding Intake Form

1. Mother's name _____

2. Baby's name _____

3. Phone number _____

4. Pediatrician _____

5. Baby's birthdate _____

6. Baby's birth weight_____

7. Current weight _____

8. Number of feedings in 24 hours _____

9. Formula use (yes/no)_____

10. Pacifier use (yes/no) _____

SELF-DIRECTED EVALUATION
SPANISH FOR BREASTFEEDING SUPPORT

TITLE: CHAPTER 5

L-CERPs: 1.3

Location:

Date:

Purpose of the activity: To help breastfeeding support professionals effectively support breastfeeding mothers in Spanish.

Please complete this evaluation questionnaire. Your anonymous responses will be used to revise this activity and to plan for future educational activities. Circle the number that best fits your evaluation of this activity.

1 Not at all   2 Somewhat   3 Almost completely   4 Completely

1. Rate your achievement of these objectives:				
a. Understand and use vocabulary and phrases related to milk supply	1	2	3	4
b. Describe things happening in the immediate present	1	2	3	4
c. Use *saber* and *conocer* and understand the difference	1	2	3	4
d. Make polite recommendations and suggestions	1	2	3	4
2. Rate the effectiveness of teaching/learning resources.	1	2	3	4
3. Were the objectives relevant to the overall purpose?	1	2	3	4
4. Was the material new to you?	1	2	3	4
5. Will you be able to use this information in your work setting?	1	2	3	4

6. How many independent study modules have you completed? _____

7. Are you interested in completing more ISMs?   ___ yes ___ no

8. How long did it take you to complete this module? _____ hours _____ minutes

9. Comments on the module. If you answered 1 to any of the above, please comment:

CHAPTER 6 ANSWER SHEET
SPANISH FOR BREASTFEEDING SUPPORT

Name:

Need help with these exercises? Looking for more opportunities to practice? Visit www.spanishforbreastfeedingsupport.com for support and additional resources to help you learn to provide breastfeeding support in Spanish.

EXERCISE 1

1. _____
2. _____
3. _____
4. _____
5. _____

EXERCISE 2

1. _____
_____
_____

2. _____
_____
_____

3. _____
_____
_____

EXERCISE 3

1. _____
2. _____
3. _____

EXERCISE 4

1. _____
2. _____
3. _____

EXERCISE 5

1. _____
2. _____
3. _____
4. _____
5. _____

CHAPTER 6 ANSWER SHEET, PAGE 2
SPANISH FOR BREASTFEEDING SUPPORT

EXERCISE 6

1. _____

2. _____

3. _____

4. _____

EXERCISE 7

Breastfeeding Intake Form

1. Mother's name _____

2. Baby's name _____

3. Phone number _____

4. Pediatrician _____

5. Baby's birthdate _____

6. Baby's birth weight_____

7. Current weight_____

8. Number of feedings in 24 hours_____

9. Number of wet diapers in 24 hours_____

10. Number of dirty diapers in 24 hours_____

11. Color of dirty diapers _____

12. Formula use (yes/no)_____

13. Pacifier use (yes/no) _____

SELF-DIRECTED EVALUATION
SPANISH FOR BREASTFEEDING SUPPORT

TITLE: CHAPTER 6

L-CERPs: 1.0

Location:

Date:

Purpose of the activity: To help breastfeeding support professionals effectively support breastfeeding mothers in Spanish.

Please complete this evaluation questionnaire. Your anonymous responses will be used to revise this activity and to plan for future educational activities. Circle the number that best fits your evaluation of this activity.

1 Not at all   2 Somewhat   3 Almost completely   4 Completely

1. Rate your achievement of these objectives:				
a. Understand and use vocabulary and phrases related to infant growth patterns and weight gain	1	2	3	4
b. Use expressions with the word *tener*	1	2	3	4
c. Describe actions using adverbs	1	2	3	4
2. Rate the effectiveness of teaching/learning resources.	1	2	3	4
3. Were the objectives relevant to the overall purpose?	1	2	3	4
4. Was the material new to you?	1	2	3	4
5. Will you be able to use this information in your work setting?	1	2	3	4

6. How many independent study modules have you completed? _____

7. Are you interested in completing more ISMs?   __ yes ___ no

8. How long did it take you to complete this module? _____ hours _____ minutes

9. Comments on the module. If you answered 1 to any of the above, please comment:

CHAPTER 7 ANSWER SHEET
Spanish for Breastfeeding Support

Name:

Need help with these exercises? Looking for more opportunities to practice? Visit www.spanishforbreastfeedingsupport.com for support and additional resources to help you learn to provide breastfeeding support in Spanish.

EXERCISE 1

1. _____
2. _____
3. _____
4. _____
5. _____

EXERCISE 2

1. _____
2. _____
3. _____
4. _____
5. _____

EXERCISE 3

1. _____
2. _____
3. _____
4. _____
5. _____

EXERCISE 4

1. _____
2. _____
3. _____
4. _____
5. _____
6. _____

EXERCISE 5

1. _____
2. _____
3. _____
4. _____
5. _____

SELF-DIRECTED EVALUATION
SPANISH FOR BREASTFEEDING SUPPORT

TITLE: CHAPTER 7

L-CERPs: 1.0

Location:

Date:

Purpose of the activity: To help breastfeeding support professionals effectively support breastfeeding mothers in Spanish.

Please complete this evaluation questionnaire. Your anonymous responses will be used to revise this activity and to plan for future educational activities. Circle the number that best fits your evaluation of this activity.

1 Not at all   2 Somewhat   3 Almost completely   4 Completely

1. Rate your achievement of these objectives: a. Understand and use vocabulary and phrases related to common breastfeeding challenges	1	2	3	4
b. Use *ir + a* to express future plans	1	2	3	4
c. Express possession or ownership	1	2	3	4
2. Rate the effectiveness of teaching/learning resources.	1	2	3	4
3. Were the objectives relevant to the overall purpose?	1	2	3	4
4. Was the material new to you?	1	2	3	4
5. Will you be able to use this information in your work setting?	1	2	3	4

6. How many independent study modules have you completed? _____

7. Are you interested in completing more ISMs? __ yes ___ no

8. How long did it take you to complete this module? _____ hours _____ minutes

9. Comments on the module. If you answered 1 to any of the above, please comment:

CHAPTER 8 ANSWER SHEET
SPANISH FOR BREASTFEEDING SUPPORT

Name:

Need help with these exercises? Looking for more opportunities to practice? Visit www.spanishforbreastfeedingsupport.com for support and additional resources to help you learn to provide breastfeeding support in Spanish.

EXERCISE 1

1. _____
2. _____
3. _____
4. _____
5. _____

EXERCISE 2

1. _____
2. _____
3. _____
4. _____
5. _____

EXERCISE 3

1. _____
2. _____
3. _____
4. _____
5. _____
6. _____
7. _____
8. _____

EXERCISE 4

1. _____
2. _____
3. _____

EXERCISE 5

1. _____
2. _____
3. _____
4. _____
5. _____

CHAPTER 8 ANSWER SHEET, PAGE 2
SPANISH FOR BREASTFEEDING SUPPORT

EXERCISE 6

1. _____

2. _____

3. _____

4. _____

SELF-DIRECTED EVALUATION
SPANISH FOR BREASTFEEDING SUPPORT

TITLE: CHAPTER 8

L-CERPs: 1.0

Location:

Date:

Purpose of the activity: To help breastfeeding support professionals effectively support breastfeeding mothers in Spanish.

Please complete this evaluation questionnaire. Your anonymous responses will be used to revise this activity and to plan for future educational activities. Circle the number that best fits your evaluation of this activity.

1 Not at all   2 Somewhat   3 Almost completely   4 Completely

1. Rate your achievement of these objectives:				
a. Understand and use vocabulary and phrases related to nutrition and breastfeeding	1	2	3	4
b. Discuss single occurrences in the past	1	2	3	4
c. Use impersonal expressions	1	2	3	4
2. Rate the effectiveness of teaching/learning resources.	1	2	3	4
3. Were the objectives relevant to the overall purpose?	1	2	3	4
4. Was the material new to you?	1	2	3	4
5. Will you be able to use this information in your work setting?	1	2	3	4

6. How many independent study modules have you completed? _____

7. Are you interested in completing more ISMs? __ yes ___ no

8. How long did it take you to complete this module? _____ hours _____ minutes

9. Comments on the module. If you answered 1 to any of the above, please comment:

CHAPTER 9 ANSWER SHEET
SPANISH FOR BREASTFEEDING SUPPORT

Name:

Need help with these exercises? Looking for more opportunities to practice? Visit www.spanishforbreastfeedingsupport.com for support and additional resources to help you learn to provide breastfeeding support in Spanish.

EXERCISE 1

1. _____
2. _____
3. _____
4. _____
5. _____

EXERCISE 2

1. _____
2. _____
3. _____
4. _____

EXERCISE 3

1. _____
2. _____
3. _____
4. _____
5. _____

EXERCISE 4

1. _____
2. _____
3. _____
4. _____
5. _____

EXERCISE 5

1. _____
2. _____
3. _____
4. _____
5. _____

CHAPTER 9 ANSWER SHEET, PAGE 2
SPANISH FOR BREASTFEEDING SUPPORT

EXERCISE 6

1. _____

2. _____

3. _____

4. _____

5. _____

SELF-DIRECTED EVALUATION
SPANISH FOR BREASTFEEDING SUPPORT

TITLE: CHAPTER 9

L-CERPs: 0.9

Location:

Date:

Purpose of the activity: To help breastfeeding support professionals effectively support breastfeeding mothers in Spanish.

Please complete this evaluation questionnaire. Your anonymous responses will be used to revise this activity and to plan for future educational activities. Circle the number that best fits your evaluation of this activity.

1 Not at all   2 Somewhat   3 Almost completely   4 Completely

1. Rate your achievement of these objectives:				
a. Understand and use vocabulary and phrases related to pumping and storing breastmilk	1	2	3	4
b. Talk about ongoing activities in the past	1	2	3	4
c. Tell time and give the time of events	1	2	3	4
2. Rate the effectiveness of teaching/learning resources.	1	2	3	4
3. Were the objectives relevant to the overall purpose?	1	2	3	4
4. Was the material new to you?	1	2	3	4
5. Will you be able to use this information in your work setting?	1	2	3	4

6. How many independent study modules have you completed? _____

7. Are you interested in completing more ISMs? ___ yes ___ no

8. How long did it take you to complete this module? _____ hours _____ minutes

9. Comments on the module. If you answered 1 to any of the above, please comment:

CHAPTER 10 ANSWER SHEET
SPANISH FOR BREASTFEEDING SUPPORT

Name:

Need help with these exercises? Looking for more opportunities to practice? Visit www.spanishforbreastfeedingsupport.com for support and additional resources to help you learn to provide breastfeeding support in Spanish.

EXERCISE 1

1. _____
2. _____
3. _____
4. _____
5. _____

EXERCISE 2

1. _____
2. _____
3. _____
4. _____
5. _____

EXERCISE 3

1. _____
2. _____
3. _____
4. _____
5. _____

EXERCISE 4

1. _____
2. _____
3. _____
4. _____
5. _____

EXERCISE 5

1. _____
2. _____
3. _____
4. _____
5. _____

CHAPTER 10 ANSWER SHEET, PAGE 2
SPANISH FOR BREASTFEEDING SUPPORT

EXERCISE 6

1. _____

2. _____

3. _____

4. _____

5. _____

SELF-DIRECTED EVALUATION
SPANISH FOR BREASTFEEDING SUPPORT

TITLE: CHAPTER 10

L-CERPs: 1.0

Location:

Date:

Purpose of the activity: To help breastfeeding support professionals effectively support breastfeeding mothers in Spanish.

Please complete this evaluation questionnaire. Your anonymous responses will be used to revise this activity and to plan for future educational activities. Circle the number that best fits your evaluation of this activity.

1 Not at all   2 Somewhat   3 Almost completely   4 Completely

1. Rate your achievement of these objectives:				
a. Understand and use vocabulary and phrases related to breastfeeding and going back to work	1	2	3	4
b. Talk about things you and others have done	1	2	3	4
c. Use "this," "that," "these" or "those" to describe objects and people	1	2	3	4
2. Rate the effectiveness of teaching/learning resources.	1	2	3	4
3. Were the objectives relevant to the overall purpose?	1	2	3	4
4. Was the material new to you?	1	2	3	4
5. Will you be able to use this information in your work setting?	1	2	3	4

6. How many independent study modules have you completed? _____

7. Are you interested in completing more ISMs? ___ yes ___ no

8. How long did it take you to complete this module? _____ hours _____ minutes

9. Comments on the module. If you answered 1 to any of the above, please comment:

CHAPTER 11 ANSWER SHEET
SPANISH FOR BREASTFEEDING SUPPORT

Name:

Need help with these exercises? Looking for more opportunities to practice? Visit www.spanishforbreastfeedingsupport.com for support and additional resources to help you learn to provide breastfeeding support in Spanish.

EXERCISE 1

1. _____
2. _____
3. _____
4. _____
5. _____

EXERCISE 2

1. _____
2. _____
3. _____
4. _____
5. _____

EXERCISE 3

1. _____
2. _____
3. _____
4. _____
5. _____

EXERCISE 4

1. _____
2. _____
3. _____
4. _____
5. _____

EXERCISE 5

1. _____
2. _____
3. _____
4. _____
5. _____

CHAPTER 11 ANSWER SHEET, PAGE 2
SPANISH FOR BREASTFEEDING SUPPORT

EXERCISE 6

1. _____

2. _____

3. _____

4. _____

5. _____

EXERCISE 7

Breastfeeding Intake Form

1. Mother's name _____

2. Baby's name _____

3. Phone number _____

4. Pediatrician _____

5. Baby's birthdate _____

6. Baby's birth weight_____

7. Current weight_____

8. Number of feedings in 24 hours_____

9. Number of wet diapers in 24 hours_____

10. Number of dirty diapers in 24 hours_____

11. Color of dirty diapers _____

12. Formula use (yes/no)_____

13. Pacifier use (yes/no) _____

SELF-DIRECTED EVALUATION
SPANISH FOR BREASTFEEDING SUPPORT

TITLE: CHAPTER 11

L-CERPs: 1.2

Location:

Date:

Purpose of the activity: To help breastfeeding support professionals effectively support breastfeeding mothers in Spanish.

Please complete this evaluation questionnaire. Your anonymous responses will be used to revise this activity and to plan for future educational activities. Circle the number that best fits your evaluation of this activity.

1 Not at all   2 Somewhat   3 Almost completely   4 Completely

1. Rate your achievement of these objectives:				
a. Understand and use vocabulary and phrases related to starting complementary foods	1	2	3	4
b. Express likes and dislikes	1	2	3	4
c. Use the conditional tense to express "should"	1	2	3	4
d. Recognize common prepositions	1	2	3	4
2. Rate the effectiveness of teaching/learning resources.	1	2	3	4
3. Were the objectives relevant to the overall purpose?	1	2	3	4
4. Was the material new to you?	1	2	3	4
5. Will you be able to use this information in your work setting?	1	2	3	4

6. How many independent study modules have you completed? _____

7. Are you interested in completing more ISMs?   __ yes ___ no

8. How long did it take you to complete this module? _____ hours _____ minutes

9. Comments on the module. If you answered 1 to any of the above, please comment:

CHAPTER 12 ANSWER SHEET
SPANISH FOR BREASTFEEDING SUPPORT

Name:

Need help with these exercises? Looking for more opportunities to practice? Visit www.spanishforbreastfeedingsupport.com for support and additional resources to help you learn to provide breastfeeding support in Spanish.

EXERCISE 1

1. _____
2. _____
3. _____
4. _____
5. _____

EXERCISE 2

1. _____
2. _____
3. _____
4. _____
5. _____

EXERCISE 3

1. _____
2. _____
3. _____
4. _____
5. _____

EXERCISE 4

1. _____
2. _____
3. _____
4. _____
5. _____

EXERCISE 5

1. _____
2. _____
3. _____
4. _____
5. _____

CHAPTER 12 ANSWER SHEET, PAGE 2
SPANISH FOR BREASTFEEDING SUPPORT

EXERCISE 7

Breastfeeding Intake Form

1. Mother's name _____

2. Baby's name _____

3. Phone number _____

4. Pediatrician _____

5. Baby's birthdate _____

6. Baby's birth weight_____

7. Lowest weight _____

8. Current Weight _____

9. Number of feedings _____

10. Number of wet diapers_____

11. Number of dirty diapers_____

12. Color of dirty diapers_____

13. Medication use_____

14. Formula use _____

15. Amount _____

16. Pacifier use _____

SELF-DIRECTED EVALUATION
SPANISH FOR BREASTFEEDING SUPPORT

TITLE: CHAPTER 12

L-CERPs: 1.0

Location:

Date:

Purpose of the activity: To help breastfeeding support professionals effectively support breastfeeding mothers in Spanish.

Please complete this evaluation questionnaire. Your anonymous responses will be used to revise this activity and to plan for future educational activities. Circle the number that best fits your evaluation of this activity.

1 Not at all   2 Somewhat   3 Almost completely   4 Completely

1. Rate your achievement of these objectives:				
a. Understand and use vocabulary and phrases related to weaning	1	2	3	4
b. Talk about the future and future plans	1	2	3	4
c. Recognize and use reflexive verbs	1	2	3	4
2. Rate the effectiveness of teaching/learning resources.	1	2	3	4
3. Were the objectives relevant to the overall purpose?	1	2	3	4
4. Was the material new to you?	1	2	3	4
5. Will you be able to use this information in your work setting?	1	2	3	4

6. How many independent study modules have you completed? _____

7. Are you interested in completing more ISMs?   __ yes ___ no

8. How long did it take you to complete this module? _____ hours _____ minutes

9. Comments on the module. If you answered 1 to any of the above, please comment:

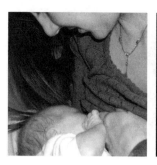

APPENDIX B

SPANISH BREASTFEEDING RESOURCES

BREASTFEEDING HELPLINES IN SPANISH

Womenshealth.gov: 1-800-994-9662

La Leche League, International: 1-877-4-LA-LECHE

BOOKS IN SPANISH

Spangler, A. 2006. *Lactancia: Guía de Consulta Para los Padres (Breastfeeding: A Parent's Guide)*. Amy's Babies.

Spangler, A. 2005. *Lactancia Materna: Sin Complicaciones (Breastfeeding Keep it Simple)*. Amy's Babies.

Ryan, R.S. & Auletta, D. 2006. *Amamantar: Un Regalo Invaluable Para tu Bebé y Para Tí (Breastfeeding: Your Priceless Gift to Your Baby and Yourself)*. Hohm Press.

Tiller, S. 2005. *Guía Fácil de Amamantar a su Bebé (Breastfeeding 101)*. TLC Publishing.

Arnold, M.A. 2003. *Guía Sobre la Lactancia Materna (Breastfeeding Care Guide)*. Care Publications, Inc.

Meek, J. Y. 2005. *Nueva Guía de Lactancia Materna (The American Academy of Pediatrics' New Mother's Guide to Breastfeeding)*. American Academy of Pediatrics.

Wiggins, P.K. 2005. *¿Por Qué Debería Amamantar a Mi Bebé? (Why Should I Nurse my Baby?)*. L.A. Publishing.

La Leche League International & Pelayo, C. 2001. *El Arte Feminino de Amamantar (The Womanly Art of Breastfeeding)*. Editorial Pax Mexico.

Rodriguez, A.M. P. 2007. *Guía Práctica para una Lactancia Exitosa* (includes DVD). Comunicadora Koine, Inc.

Wiggins, P.K. 2006. *Breastfeeding: A Mother's Gift (Spanish edition)*. L.A. Publishing.

HANDOUTS IN SPANISH

Office of Women's Health, Department of Health and Human Services. "Una Guía Fácil para la Lactancia" ("Easy Guide to Breastfeeding"). www.4woman.gov/pub/bf.cfm

UNICEF, The Baby Friendly Initiative. "Amamantar a tu Bebe" ("Breastfeeding your Baby"). www.babyfriendly.org.uk/pdfs/spanish/bfyb_spanish2.pdf

La Leche League International, tear off sheets English and Spanish, various topics. http://store.llli.org/public/category/5

Medela, Inc. Breastfeeding tear-off sheets, various topics, English and Spanish. www.medelabreastfeedingus.com/for-professionals/lc-information

Breastfeeding Task Force of Greater Los Angeles. "A Mother's 10 Steps to Successful Breastfeeding: Even if your Hospital isn't Baby Friendly" (Spanish version). www.breastfeedingtaskforla.org/10-steps/horizonal%20-%20FINAL%20Spanish.pdf

Texas Department of State Health Services. Breastfeeding handouts, various topics, English and Spanish. www.dshs.state.tx.us/wichd/bf/bfpublic.shtm

South Los Angeles Health Projects WIC Program, 2004. Breastfeeding Flyers, various topics, English and Spanish. www.breastfeedingtaskforla.org/resources/breastfeeding-public-education.htm

California Department of Public Health. Breastfeeding handouts, various topics, English and Spanish. http://ww2.cdph.ca.gov/programs/wicworks/Pages/WIC-BFResource.aspx

Hoover, K. & Wilson-Clay, B. 2003. *Diaper Diary*, Spanish version. www.ibreastfeeding.com/catalog/product_info.php?cPath=20&products_id=138

Minnesota Department of Health. Breastfeeding handouts, various topics, English and Spanish. www.health.state.mn.us/divs/fh/wic/bf/spanish.html

Childbirth Graphics. Breastfeeding tear pad set, various topics, English and Spanish. www.childbirthgraphics.com/storefrontB2CWEB/ itemdetail.do?action=prepare_detail&itm_id=25116&itm_ index=9

Wiggins, P.K. *When Disasters Happen: Breastfeeding in Emergencies.* LA Publishing. www.breastfeedingbooks.com/pages/emerg.html

Massachusetts Breastfeeding Coalition, "Making Milk is Easy!" "It's my birthday, give me a hug (skin-to-skin)," various others. www.massbfc.org

PROMOTIONAL MATERIALS IN SPANISH (POSTERS, PINS, MAGNETS, T-SHIRTS)

Childbirth Graphics: www.childbirthgraphics.com

Noodle Soup: www.noodlesoup.com

Massachusetts Breastfeeding Coalition: www.massbfc.org

VIDEOS/DVDs AVAILABLE IN SPANISH

Injoy Videos. 2008. "Better Breastfeeding: Your Guide to a Healthy Start." www.injoyvideos.com

Eagle Video Productions. 2006. "Breastfeeding and Returning to Work," www.eaglevideo.com

Mother of 7, Inc. 2008. "Mother of 7 Breastfeeding Basics & FAQ Multi-lingual DVD." www.motherof7.com

Eagle Video Productions. 2008. "Breastfeeding: What's a Dad Supposed to Do?" www.eaglevideo.com

Injoy Videos. 2000. "14 Steps to Better Breastfeeding." www.injoyvideos.com

LA Publishing. 2007. "Breastfeeding: You Can Do It!" www.breastfeedingbooks.com

Texas Department of State Health Services. 2006. "To Baby with Love / The Comfortable Latch." www.dshs.state. tx.us/wichd/bf/videos.shtm

Injoy Videos. 1998. "Breastfeeding: The Natural Choice (teens)." www.injoyvideos.com

Geddes Productions. 1992. "Delivery Self Attachment (DVD)." www.geddesproduction.com

Newman, J. & Kennerman, E. 2007. "Dr. Jack Newman's Visual Guide to Breastfeeding" (Spanish subtitles). www.ibreastfeeding.com

Geddes Productions. 2005. "Método Madre Canguro, (Kangaroo Mother Care) DVD." www.geddesproduction.com

Vida Health Communications., 1998. "Breastfeeding: How to, Why to." www.vida-health.com

CHILDREN'S BOOKS IN SPANISH

Newman, C. 2006. *Cerca del Corazón de Mamá (Near Mama's Heart).* Trafford Publishing.

Martin, C. & Rainey, S. 1994. *Nos Gusta Amamantar (We Like to Nurse).* Hohm Press.

La Leche League, International. www.llli.org/LangEspanol.html

Minnesota Department of Health. www.health.state.mn.us/divs/fh/wic/spanish/spindex.html

TRAINING MATERIALS IN SPANISH

USDA Food and Nutrition Services. "Loving Support through Peer Counseling" training materials in Spanish: Power Point presentation, curriculum modules, handouts, reproducibles. http://www.nal.usda.gov/wicworks/ Learning_Center/support_peer_training05sp.html

SPANISH TOOLS FOR BREASTFEEDING SUPPORT PEOPLE

International Lactation Consultant Association. 2004. "Spanish Breastfeeding Glossary," laminated. http://www.ilca.org/i4a/ams/amsstore/category.cfm?category_id=9

"Spanish Pocket Guide for Breastfeeding Support." www.childbirthgraphics.com

Healthtranslations.com. www.healthtranslations.com

MEDICAL SPANISH TEXTBOOKS

Ortega, P. 2006. *Spanish and the Medical Interview: A Textbook for Clinically Relevant Medical Spanish.* Saunders.

Rios, J. & Fernandez, J. 2004. *Complete Medical Spanish: A Practical Course for Quick and Confident Communication.* McGraw-Hill.

Jarvis, A.C. & Lebredo, R. 2000. *Spanish for Medical Personnel.* Houghton Mifflin Company.

MEDICAL SPANISH WEBSITES

Medical Spanish for Health Professionals
http://www.123teachme.com/learn_spanish/medical-spanish

A Translation Handguide For Spanish-English Medical Terminology
http://www.auburn.edu/forlang/Spanish/Medical_terms/

Medical Spanish for Healthcare Providers
http://www.practicingspanish.com/index.html

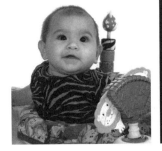

APPENDIX C

ENGLISH-SPANISH GLOSSARY

a little	poco
a lot	mucho
about	acerca de
abscess	abceso (m.)
according to, in accordance with	de acuerdo con
accustom oneself, to; get used to, to	acostumbrarse
aches, pains	dolores (m.)
adjust, to	ajustar
adopted	adoptado
adoptive nursing	lactancia adoptiva (f.)
advice	consejos (m.)
affect, to	afectar
affection	cariños (m.)
again	otra vez
against, next to	contra
alcohol	alcohol (m.)
alcoholic beverage	bebida alcohólica (f.)
allergy	alergia (f.)
alleviate, to	aliviar
also	también
alveoli	alvéolos (m.)
alveolus	alvéolo (m.)
always	siempre
American Academy of Pediatrics	Academia Americana de Pediatría (f.)
amount	cantidad (f.)
anemia	anemia (f.)
antibiotics	antibióticos (m.)
any	cualquier
appointment	cita (f.)
approximately	aproximadamente
arch, to	arquear
area	área (f.)
areola	areola (f.)
arm	brazo (m.)
asymmetrical latch	enganche asimétrico (m.)
at birth	al nacer
at least	al menos
at, in	en
attach, to (to the breast)	prenderse

B

attend, to	asistir
augmentation surgery	cirugía de aumento mamario (f.)
aunt	tía (f.)
avocado	aguacate (m.)
avoid, to	evitar
baby	bebé (m./f.)
baby blues	depresión posparto (f.), melancolía de maternidad (f.)
baby bottle	mamadera (f.), biberón (m.)
back (anatomy)	espalda (f.)
back (position)	atrás
balanced	balanceado
bare, naked	descubierto
be able, to	poder
be pleasing, to	gustar
bed	cama (f.)
begin, to	comenzar
believe, to	creer
better, best	mejor
big	grande
bilirubin	bilirrubina (f.)
birth	nacimiento (m.)
birth control	control de natalidad (m.)
birth control pill	pastilla anticonceptiva (f.)
birth weight	peso al nacer (m.)
biting, to bite	morder
bleb (milk blister)	ampolla (f.)
bleeding, to bleed	sangrar
blister	ampolla (f.)
blood	sangre (f.)
body	cuerpo (m.)
bonding	creación de lazos afectivos (f.)
book	libro (m.)
boss	jefe (m.)
bottle	biberón (m.)
bottle-fed	alimentado con biberón
bottle-feeding, to bottle-feed	alimentar con biberón
bowel movement	excremento (m.), evacuación (f.)
bowl	tazón (m.)
bowl of warm water, double boiler	baño María (m.), tazón de agua tibia (m.)
bra	brassiere, sostén (m.)
break, rest	descanso (m.)
breast augmentation surgery	cirugía de aumento mamario (f.)
breast implant	implante mamario (m.)
breast infection	infección del pecho (f.)
breast massage	masaje del pecho (m.)
breast pads	almohadillas de lactancia (f.)
breast pump	sacaleches (m.), bomba (f.), tiraleches (m.)
breast reduction surgery	cirugía de reducción mamaria (f.)
breast refusal	rechazo del pecho (m.)
breast shells	conchas protectoras (f.)

C

breast, chest	pecho, seno (m.)
breastfeed, to; nurse, to	amamantar, dar pecho
breastfeeding	lactancia (f.)
breastfeeding	lactancia materna (f.)
breastfeeding in public	amamantar en público
breastfeeding support group	grupo de apoyo a la lactancia (m.)
breastmilk	leche materna (f.)
breastmilk donation	donación de leche materna (f.)
bring close, to	acercar
brother	hermano (m.)
burning sensation	ardor (m.)
burp your baby, to	sacarle el gas al bebé
burp, to	eructar
but	pero
button	botón (m.)
cabbage leaves	hojas de col (f.)
Caesarean section	cesárea (f.)
calcium	calcio (m.)
call, to (by phone)	llamar
cancer	cáncer (m.)
cause, to	causar
cc	cc o cm³ (centímetro cúbico) (m.)
cereal	cereal (m.)
certain	cierto
challenge	reto (m.)
change	cambio (m.)
change, to	cambiar
chart, file	expediente (m.)
chat, to	platicar
child	niño (m.)/niña (f.)
childbirth	nacimiento, parto (m.)
chili pepper	chile (m.)
chills	escalofríos (m.)
chin	barbilla (f.)
chiropractic treatment	tratamiento quiropráctico (m.)
choke, to	atorarse
cigarette	cigarrillo (m.)
circumcision	circuncisión (f.)
cleft lip	labio leporino (m.)
cleft palate	paladar hendido (m.)
clenching, to clench	apretar la mandíbula
clicking sounds	sonidos de chasquidos (m.)
clinic	clínica (f.)
clock, watch	reloj (m.)
close	cerca
close contact	contacto cercano (m.)
cluster feeding	períodos de alimentación frecuente (m.)
coffee	café (m.)
cold (illness)	resfriado (m.)
cold compress	compresa fría (f.)
colostrum	calostro (m.)

come down, to; let down, to	bajar
come off, to; take off, to	quitarse
comfort	consuelo (m.)
comfortable	cómodo
coming in (milk)	subida de la leche (f.)
consult, to	consultar
continue, to	continuar
continue, to; follow, to	seguir
contraception	anticonceptivo (m.)
control, to	controlar
correct	cierto, correcto
co-sleeping	colecho (m.)
counselor	consejera (f.)
cousin	primo (m.)
crack (drug)	metanfetamina (f.)
cradle hold	posición de cuna (f.)
crib	cuna (f.)
cross-cradle hold	posición de cuna cruzada (f.)
crying, to cry	llorar
cuddle, to	acurrucar
culture	cultura (f.)
cup	taza (f.), vaso (m.)
dairy	productos lácteos (m.)
dangerous	peligroso
date (calendar)	fecha (f.)
daughter	hija (f.)
day	día (m.)
daycare	guardería (f.)
dehydration	deshidratación (f.)
demonstrate, to	demostrar
depend on, to	depender de
depression	depresión (f.)
diabetes	diabetes (f.)
dial	regulador (m.)
diaper	pañal, pamper (m.)
diaper rash	pañalitis (f.)
diarrhea	diarrea (f.)
diet	dieta (f.)
difference	diferencia (f.)
difficult	difícil
dirty	sucio
dirty diaper	pañal sucio (m.)
dishwasher	lavaplatos (m.)
distract, to	distraer
do not use	no usar
do, to; make, to	hacer
doctor	doctor, médico (m.)
donated milk	leche donada (f.)
Down Syndrome	síndrome de Down (m.)
drink, to	tomar
dropper	gotero (m.)
drugs	drogas (f.)

D

each	cada
ear (inside)	oído (m.)
ear (outside)	oreja (f.)
ear infection	infección del oído (f.)
eat, to	comer
eczema	eccema (m.)
eliminate, to	eliminar
elimination diet	dieta de eliminacion (f.)
embarassed	avergonzado
employer	empleador, patrón (m.)
English	inglés (m.)
engorged, swollen	hinchado
engorgement	hinchazón (m.)
enough	suficiente
estrogen	estrógeno (m.)
excellent	excelente
excess lipase	exceso de lipasa (m.)
exclusive	exclusivo
exclusive breastfeeding	lactancia exclusiva (f.)
exercise	ejercicio (m.)
explain, to	explicar
explore, to	explorar
express, to; pump, to	sacarse (la leche)
extended breastfeeding	lactancia prolongada (f.)
failure to thrive	retraso del crecimiento (m.)
fall asleep, to	dormirse
family	familia (f.)
fast	rápido
fat (noun)	grasa (f.)
father	padre, papá (m.)
feed on cue, to; to feed on demand	alimentar a demanda
feed, to	alimentar
feeding	toma (f.), comida de pecho (f.), lactada (f.)
feel, to (an emotion)	sentir, sentirse
feeling	sentimiento (m.)
fenugreek	fenogreco (m.)
fever	fiebre (f.)
finger	dedo (m.)
finger-feeding	alimentación con el dedo (f.)
finish, to	terminar
first	primer, primero
fish	pez (m.)
flange	copa de succión (f.)
flat nipples	pezones planos (m.)
flow	flujo (m.)
flu, cold	gripe (f.)
fluid, liquid	líquido (m.)
football hold	posición de fútbol americano/sandía/lateral debajo del brazo (f.)
forceful let-down	bajada fuerte (f.)

foremilk	leche inicial (f.)
formula	fórmula (f.)
freezer	congelador (m.)
freezing, to freeze	congelar
frenulum	frenillo (m.)
frequency	frecuencia (f.)
friend	amigo (m.), amiga (f.)
fruit	fruta (f.)
frustrated	frustrado
full	lleno
fun, to have	divertirse
fussy	inquieto
gain weight, to; increase, to	aumentar, subir de peso

G

galactocele	galactocele (m.)
galactogogue	galactogogo (m.)
gas	gases (m.)
gassy	que causa gases
gently	suavemente
give, to	dar
glossary	glosario (m.)
good	bueno
good afternoon	buenas tardes
good evening	buenas noches
good morning	buenos días
goodbye	adiós
gradually	poco a poco
grain	grano (m.)
grandchild	nieto (m.), nieta (f.)
grandfather	abuelo (m.)
grandmother	abuela (f.)
green	verde
grow, to	crecer
growth	crecimiento (m.)
growth spurt	estirón (m.)
gulping, to gulp	tragar
gum	encía (f.)
hand	mano (f.)

H

hand express, to	extraer la leche a mano
happen, to; occur, to	pasar, ocurrir
have, to	tener
head	cabeza (f.)
heal oneself, to	curarse
health	salud (f.)
healthy	sano, saludable
hear, to	oír
heat	calor (m.)
heat up, to	calentar
heavy	pesado
hello, hi	hola
help, to	ayudar
hemorrhage	hemorragia (f.)

herb	hierba (f.)
here	aquí
hindmilk	leche final (f.)
hip	cadera (f.)
HIV virus	virus VIH (m.)
hold	posición (f.)
hold, to	sostener
hormone	hormona (f.)
hospital	hospital (m.)
hot, spicy	picante
hour	hora (f.)
how long	cuánto tiempo
how many	cuántos
how many times	cuántas veces
how much	cuánto
how often	con qué frecuencia
hungry, to be	tener hambre
hurt, to	doler
husband	esposo (m.)
hypertension	hipertensión (f.)
hyperthyroidism	hipertiroidismo (m.)
hypoglycemia	hipoglicemia (f.)
ice	hielo (m.)
if, whether	si
implants	implantes mamarios (m.)
important	importante
increase, to	incrementar
infected	infectado
injury	herida (f.)
insert, to	insertar
insulin	insulina (f.)
interest	interés (m.)
introduce, to	introducir
inverted nipples	pezones invertidos (m.)
iron	hierro (m.)
it's important	es importante
it's necessary	es necesario
jaundice	bilirrubina, ictericia (f.)
jaw	mandíbula (f.)
Kangaroo Care	cuidado del canguro (m.)
keep, to; store, to	guardar
know, to (a fact)	saber
know, to (to be familiar with)	conocer
La Leche League, International	La Liga de la Leche, Internacional (f.)
lactation consultant	consultora de lactancia (f.)
lactation counselor	consejera de lactancia (f.)
lactational amenorrhea method	método de amenorea lactacional (m.)
large	grande
large breasts	senos grandes (m.)
last, to; take a long time, to	durar
latch	enganche (m.), agarre (m.)

I, J, K

L

M

latch onto, to	pegarse al pecho, agarrar, prenderse
later	más tarde
law	ley (f.)
leader	líder (m./f.)
leaking milk	goteo de leche (m.)
leaking, to leak	gotear
leave, to; let, to	dejar
let down, to (milk)	bajar
letdown	reflejo de eyección de la leche (m.), bajada (f.)
lethargic	letárgico
like before	como antes
lips	labios (m.)
listen, to; hear, to	escuchar
long	largo
look at, to	mirar
look for, to; seek, to	buscar
look like, to	parecer
losing weight, to lose weight	perder peso, rebajar
lump in breast	bulto en el pecho (m.)
lunch	almuerzo (m.)
maintain, to	mantener
majority, most	mayoría (f.)
make milk, to	producir leche
mammogram	mamografía (m.)
manual expression	expresión manual (f.)
mashed	machacado
massage	masaje (m.)
massage, to	masajear
mastitis	mastitis (f.)
maternity leave	licencia de maternidad (f.)
mean, to	significar
meconium	meconio (m.)
medication	medicamento (m.), medicina (f.)
menstrual period	período menstrual (m.), regla (f.)
microwave	microondas (m.)
milk	leche (f.)
milk ducts	conductos lácteos (m.)
milk supply	cantidad de leche (f.)
milliliter (ml)	mililitro (m.)
mix, to	mezclar
Montgomery glands	glándulas de Montgomery (f.)
month	mes (m.)
more than	más que
mostly, mainly	principalmente
mother	madre, mamá (f.)
mother-in-law	suegra (f.)
mouth	boca (f.)
movement	movimiento (m.)
multiples	múltiples (m.)

named, to be	llamarse
necessary	necesario
neck	cuello (m.)
need, to	necesitar
nephew	sobrino (m.)
newborn	recién nacido (m.)
next	próximo
NICU (Neonatal Intensive Care Unit)	unidad de cuidados intensivos neonatal (f.)
niece	sobrina (f.)
night	noche (f.)
night feedings	tomas nocturnas (f.)
nipple	pezón (m.)
nipple cream	crema para pezones (f.)
nipple shield	pezonera (f.)
none, no	ningún
normal	normal
normally, usually	normalmente
nose	nariz (f.)
nose to nipple	nariz contra el pezón
now	ahora
number	número (m.)
nurse (person)	enfermera (f.)
nurse, to	dar pecho
nursery (hospital)	sala de recién nacidos (f.)
nursing bra	brassiere/sostén para la lactancia (m.)
nursing pads	almohadillas de lactancia (f.)
nursing pillow	cojín de lactancia (m.)
nursing strike	huelga de lactancia (f.)
nutritionist	nutricionista (m./f.)
nutritious	nutritivo

obesity	obesidad (f.)
obligate, to; force, to; require, to	obligar
offer, to	ofrecer
office	oficina (f.)
only, just	sólo
open, to	abrir
other	otro
ounce	onza (f.)
oversupply	sobreproducción de leche (f.)
own (adj.)	propio
oxytocin	oxitocina (f.)
pacifier	chupón (m.)
pain	dolor (m.)
paper	papel (m.)
parents	padres (m.)
partner, a pair	pareja (f.)
parts	piezas (f.)
pay, to	pagar
pediatrician	pediatra (m./f.)
people	gente (f.)

perfect	perfecto
pierced nipples	pezones perforados (m.)
pillow	almohada (f.)
place in cradle hold, to	acunar
placenta	placenta (f.)
plantain	plátano (m.)
plastic	plástico
play, to	jugar
please	por favor
plug	tapón (m.)
plugged duct	conducto lácteo obstruido (m.)
polycystic ovary syndrome (PCOS)	síndrome de ovario policístico (m.)
pork	puerco (m.)
position	posición (f.)
position, to; place, to	colocar
postpartum depression	depresión posparto (f.)
pound	libra (f.)
practice	práctica (f.)
pregnancy	embarazo (m.)
pregnant	embarazada
premature	prematuro
prepare oneself, to	prepararse
pressure	presión (f.)
probably	probablemente
problem	problema (m.)
produce, to	producir
progesterone	progesterona (f.)
prolactin	prolactina (f.)
protein	proteína (f.)
pump, to	extraer, sacarse la leche, bombear
pumping	extracción (f.)
pureed	puré de (m.), en forma de puré
put, to; place, to	poner
quality	calidad (f.)
quantity	cantidad (f.)
question	pregunta (f.)
quickly	rápidamente
quite a bit, a lot	bastante
rash	ronchas (f.), salpullido (m.), sarpullido (m.)
Raynaud's Phenomenon	fenómeno de Raynaud (m.)
react, to	reaccionar
reaction	reacción (f.)
ready	listo
receive, to	recibir
recommend, to	recomendar
red	rojo
reduce, to; lower, to	reducir
refrigerator	refrigerador (m.)
regularly	regularmente
relactation	relactación (f.), relactancia (f.)

Q

R

rent, to	alquilar, rentar
rented	alquilado
repeat, to	repetir
repositioning baby	reposicionar al bebé
rest, to	descansar
retracted nipples	pezones retraídos, pezones hundidos (m.)
return	regreso (m.)
return, to; go back, to	regresar
rich	rico
room temperature	temperatura ambiente (f.)
same	mismo
sandwich	emparedado, sándwich (m.)
say, to	decir
scheduling	programación de comidas, imposición de un horario (f.)
second	segundo
seek, to	buscar
Sheehan's Syndrome	síndrome de Sheehan (m.)
should, must	deber
shoulder	hombro (m.)
show, to; teach, to	enseñar
sick	enfermo
side lying hold	posición de lado (f.)
SIDS (Sudden Infant Death Syndrome)	síndrome de muerte infantil súbita (SMIS) (m.)
simply	simplemente
sister	hermana (f.)
sister-in-law	cuñada (f.)
sit, to; sit down, to	sentarse
size	tamaño
skin	piel (f.)
skin-to-skin	piel con piel
sleep, to	dormir
sleepy	cansado
sling	cargador (m.)
slow	lento, despacio
slowly	lentamente
small	pequeño
smoking, to smoke	fumar
so (so long)	tan
so much	tanto
soapy smell	olor a jabón (m.)
solid food	alimentos sólidos (m.)
solution	solución (f.)
something	algo
sometimes	a veces
son	hijo (m.)
soon	pronto
sore	adolorido
sore nipples	pezones adoloridos (m.)
sound	sonido (m.)

soy	soya (f.)
Spanish	español (m.)
special	especial
special needs	necesidades especiales (f.)
speed	velocidad (f.)
spit up, to	regurgitar, escupir
spoon	cuchara (f.)
squeeze, to	apretar
stain, spot	mancha (f.)
start, to	comenzar, empezar
stay, to	quedar
sterilization	esterilización (f.)
still, yet	todavía
stomach	estómago (m.)
stool (furniture)	taburete (m.)
storage	almacenamiento (m.)
storage bags	bolsas para almacenar (f.)
straight line	línea recta (f.)
success	éxito (m.)
suck, to; suction, to	succionar
sucking bursts	períodos de succión rápida (m.)
suckling	mamar
suction	succión (f.)
sufficient	suficiente
suggest, to	sugerir
suggestion	sugerencia (f.)
sunk into	hundido
supplement, to	suplementar
supplemental feeding	alimentación suplementaria (f.)
supplemental nursing system	sistema de lactancia suplementaria (m.)
supplements	suplementos (m.)
supply and demand	oferta y demanda
supply, back-up	provisión (f.)
supply, milk supply	cantidad de leche (f.)
surgery	cirugía (f.)
swallow, to	tragar
sweet potato	camote (m.)
symptom	síntoma (m.)
system	sistema (m.)
tablespoon	cucharada (f.)
take off, to (the breast)	desprender, quitar
take, to; drink, to	tomar
take, to; wear, to	llevar
talk, to; speak, to	hablar
tandem nursing	lactancia en tándem (dos bebés) (f.)
teaspoon	cucharadita (f.)
technique	técnica (f.)
teeth	dientes (m.)
teething	dentición (f.)
telephone	teléfono (m.)
telephone number	número de teléfono (m.)

tender	tierno
thank you	gracias
that	eso
thawing, to thaw	descongelar
then	entonces
thirsty, to be	tener sed
this	este
throwing up	vomitar
thrush	infección de hongo (f.), algodoncillo (m.)
tilt back, to	inclinarse hacia atrás
time (chronological)	tiempo
time, times (occurrences)	vez, veces (f.)
tired	cansado
today	hoy
toddler	niño pequeño (m.)
toddler nursing	amamantar al niño pequeño
together	juntos
tongue	lengua (f.)
tongue tie	frenillo corto (m.), anquiloglosia (f.)
too much	demasiado
touch, to	tocar
traditional Mexican drink	atole (m.)
triplets	trillizos (m.)
true	verdad (f.)
try, to	intentar, tratar de
tubing (for pump)	tubería (f.)
tummy	panza (f.), barriga (f.)
tummy-to-tummy	panza con panza
twins	gemelos, mellizos (m.)
uncle	tío (m.)
understand, to	entender
underwire	sostén con varillas, sostén con aros (m.)
until	hasta
uphill (nursing position)	posición vertical (f.)
upset	inquieto, molesto
urine	orina (f.)
use, to	usar
utilize, to	utilizar
vaccination, vaccine	vacuna (f.)
vasospasm	vasospasmo (m.)
vegetable	vegetal (m.)
very	muy
Vitamin D	Vitamina D (f.)
vomiting, to vomit	vomitar
wake, to	despertarse
want, to	querer
warm	tibia
warm compress	compresa caliente (f.)
wash, to; clean, to	lavar
waste, to	desperdiciar

U, V, W

watch, clock	reloj (m.)
water	agua (m.)
wean, to	destetar
weaned	destetado
weaning	destete (m.)
wear, to; take, to	llevar
weigh, to	pesar
weight	peso (m.)
weight gain	ganancia de peso (f.)
weight loss	pérdida de peso (f.)
welcome	bienvenidos
wet	mojado
wet compress	compresa mojada (f.)
wet diaper	pañal mojado (m.)
wheat	trigo (m.)
white	blanco
WIC	WIC
wide	ancho, amplio
wife	esposa (f.)
wish, to; want, to	desear
work	trabajo (m.)
worried	preocupado
worry, to	preocuparse
yawn	bostezo (m.)
year	año (m.)
yeast infection	infección de hongo (f.)
yellow	amarillo
yes	sí
yesterday	ayer
you're welcome	de nada

Y

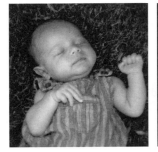

APPENDIX D

SPANISH-ENGLISH GLOSSARY

a veces	sometimes
abceso (m.)	abscess
abrir	open, to
abuela (f.)	grandmother
abuelo (m.)	grandfather
Academia Americana de Pediatría (f.)	American Academy of Pediatrics
acerca de	about
acercar	bring close, to
acostumbrarse	accustom oneself, to; get used to, to
acunar	place in cradle hold, to
acurrucar	cuddle, to
adiós	goodbye
adolorido	sore
adoptado	adopted
afectar	affect, to
agua (m.)	water
aguacate (m.)	avocado
ahora	now
ajustar	adjust, to
al menos	at least
al nacer	at birth
alcohol (m.)	alcohol
alergia (f.)	allergy
algo	something
alimentación con el dedo (f.)	finger-feeding
alimentación suplementaria (f.)	supplemental feeding
alimentado con biberón	bottle-fed
alimentar	feed, to
alimentar a demanda	feed on cue, to; to feed on demand
alimentar con biberón	bottle-feeding, to bottle-feed
alimentos sólidos (m.)	solid food
aliviar	alleviate, to
almacenamiento (m.)	storage
almohada (f.)	pillow
almohadillas de lactancia (f.)	breast pads
almohadillas de lactancia (f.)	nursing pads

almuerzo (m.)	lunch
alquilado	rented
alquilar, rentar	rent, to
alvéolo (m.)	alveolus
alvéolos (m.)	alveoli
amamantar al niño pequeño	toddler nursing
amamantar en público	breastfeeding in public
amamantar, dar pecho	breastfeed, to; nurse, to
amarillo	yellow
amigo (m.), amiga (f.)	friend
ampolla (f.)	bleb (milk blister)
ampolla (f.)	blister
ancho, amplio	wide
anemia (f.)	anemia
año (m.)	year
antibióticos (m.)	antibiotics
anticonceptivo (m.)	contraception
apretar	squeeze, to
apretar la mandíbula	clenching, to clench
aproximadamente	approximately
aquí	here
ardor (m.)	burning sensation
área (f.)	area
areola (f.)	areola
arquear	arch, to
asistir	attend, to
atole (m.)	traditional Mexican drink
atorarse	choke, to
atrás	back (position)
aumentar, subir de peso	gain weight, to; increase, to
avergonzado	embarassed
ayer	yesterday
ayudar	help, to
bajada fuerte (f.)	forceful let-down
bajar	come down, to; let down, to
bajar	let down, to (milk)
balanceado	balanced
baño María (m.), tazón de agua tibia (m.)	bowl of warm water, double boiler
barbilla (f.)	chin
bastante	quite a bit, a lot
bebé (m./f.)	baby
bebida alcohólica (f.)	alcoholic beverage
biberón (m.)	bottle
bienvenidos	welcome
bilirrubina, ictericia (f.)	jaundice
bilirrubina (f.)	bilirubin
blanco	white
boca (f.)	mouth
bolsas para almacenar (f.)	storage bags
bostezo (m.)	yawn
botón (m.)	button

B

C

brassiere, sostén (m.)	bra
brassiere/sostén para la lactancia (m.)	nursing bra
brazo (m.)	arm
buenas noches	good evening
buenas tardes	good afternoon
bueno	good
buenos días	good morning
bulto en el pecho (m.)	lump in breast
buscar	look for, to; seek, to
buscar	seek, to
cabeza (f.)	head
cada	each
cadera (f.)	hip
café (m.)	coffee
calcio (m.)	calcium
calentar	heat up, to
calidad (f.)	quality
calor (m.)	heat
calostro (m.)	colostrum
cama (f.)	bed
cambiar	change, to
cambio (m.)	change
camote (m.)	sweet potato
cáncer (m.)	cancer
cansado	sleepy
cansado	tired
cantidad (f.)	amount
cantidad (f.)	quantity
cantidad de leche (f.)	milk supply
cantidad de leche (f.)	supply, milk supply
cargador (m.)	sling
cariños (m.)	affection
causar	cause, to
cc o cm³ (centímetro cúbico) (m.)	cc
cerca	close
cereal (m.)	cereal
cesárea (f.)	Caesarean section
chile (m.)	chili pepper
chupón (m.)	pacifier
cierto	certain
cierto, correcto	correct
cigarrillo (m.)	cigarette
circuncisión (f.)	circumcision
cirugía (f.)	surgery
cirugía de aumento mamario (f.)	augmentation surgery
cirugía de aumento mamario (f.)	breast augmentation surgery
cirugía de reducción mamaria (f.)	breast reduction surgery
cita (f.)	appointment
clínica (f.)	clinic
cojín de lactancia (m.)	nursing pillow
colecho (m.)	co-sleeping

colocar	position, to; place, to
comenzar	begin, to
comenzar, empezar	start, to
comer	eat, to
como antes	like before
cómodo	comfortable
compresa caliente (f.)	warm compress
compresa fría (f.)	cold compress
compresa mojada (f.)	wet compress
con qué frecuencia	how often
conchas protectoras (f.)	breast shells
conducto lácteo obstruido (m.)	plugged duct
conductos lácteos (m.)	milk ducts
congelador (m.)	freezer
congelar	freezing, to freeze
conocer	know, to (to be familiar with)
consejera (f.)	counselor
consejera de lactancia (f.)	lactation counselor
consejos (m.)	advice
consuelo (m.)	comfort
consultar	consult, to
consultora de lactancia (f.)	lactation consultant
contacto cercano (m.)	close contact
continuar	continue, to
contra	against, next to
control de natalidad (m.)	birth control
controlar	control, to
copa de succión (f.)	flange
creación de lazos afectivos (f.)	bonding
crecer	grow, to
crecimiento (m.)	growth
creer	believe, to
crema para pezones (f.)	nipple cream
cualquier	any
cuántas veces	how many times
cuánto	how much
cuánto tiempo	how long
cuántos	how many
cuchara (f.)	spoon
cucharada (f.)	tablespoon
cucharadita (f.)	teaspoon
cuello (m.)	neck
cuerpo (m.)	body
cuidado del canguro (m.)	Kangaroo Care
cultura (f.)	culture
cuna (f.)	crib
cuñada (f.)	sister-in-law
curarse	heal oneself, to
dar	give, to
dar pecho	nurse, to
de acuerdo con	according to, in accordance with

D

de nada	you're welcome
deber	should, must
decir	say, to
dedo (m.)	finger
dejar	leave, to; let, to
demasiado	too much
demostrar	demonstrate, to
dentición (f.)	teething
depender de	depend on, to
depresión (f.)	depression
depresión posparto (f.)	postpartum depression
depresión posparto (f.), melancolía de maternidad (f.)	baby blues
descansar	rest, to
descanso (m.)	break, rest
descongelar	thawing, to thaw
descubierto	bare, naked
desear	wish, to; want, to
deshidratación (f.)	dehydration
desperdiciar	waste, to
despertarse	wake, to
desprender, quitar	take off, to (the breast)
destetado	weaned
destetar	wean, to
destete (m.)	weaning
día (m.)	day
diabetes (f.)	diabetes
diarrea (f.)	diarrhea
dientes (m.)	teeth
dieta (f.)	diet
dieta de eliminacion (f.)	elimination diet
diferencia (f.)	difference
dificil	difficult
distraer	distract, to
divertirse	fun, to have
doctor, médico (m.)	doctor
doler	hurt, to
dolor (m.)	pain
dolores (m.)	aches, pains
donación de leche materna (f.)	breastmilk donation
dormir	sleep, to
dormirse	fall asleep, to
drogas (f.)	drugs
durar	last, to; take a long time, to
eccema (m.)	eczema
ejercicio (m.)	exercise
eliminar	eliminate, to
embarazada	pregnant
embarazo (m.)	pregnancy
emparedado, sándwich (m.)	sandwich
empleador, patrón (m.)	employer

E

en	at, in
encía (f.)	gum
enfermera (f.)	nurse (person)
enfermo	sick
enganche (m.), agarre (m.)	latch
enganche asimétrico (m.)	asymmetrical latch
enseñar	show, to; teach, to
entender	understand, to
entonces	then
eructar	burp, to
es importante	it's important
es necesario	it's necessary
escalofríos (m.)	chills
escuchar	listen, to; hear, to
eso	that
espalda (f.)	back (anatomy)
español (m.)	Spanish
especial	special
esposa (f.)	wife
esposo (m.)	husband
este	this
esterilización (f.)	sterilization
estirón (m.)	growth spurt
estómago (m.)	stomach
estrógeno (m.)	estrogen
evitar	avoid, to
excelente	excellent
exceso de lipasa (m.)	excess lipase
exclusivo	exclusive
excremento (m.), evacuación (f.)	bowel movement
éxito (m.)	success
expediente (m.)	chart, file
explicar	explain, to
explorar	explore, to
expresión manual (f.)	manual expression
extracción (f.)	pumping
extraer la leche a mano	hand express, to
extraer, sacarse la leche, bombear	pump, to
familia (f.)	family
fecha (f.)	date
fenogreco (m.)	fenugreek
fenómeno de Raynaud (m.)	Raynaud's Phenomenon
fiebre (f.)	fever
flujo (m.)	flow
fórmula (f.)	formula
frecuencia (f.)	frequency
frenillo (m.)	frenulum
frenillo corto (m.); anquiloglosia (f.)	tongue tie
frustrado	frustrated
fruta (f.)	fruit
fumar	smoking, to smoke

F

G

galactocele (m.)	galactocele
galactogogo (m.)	galactogogue
ganancia de peso (f.)	weight gain
gases (m.)	gas
gemelos, mellizos (m.)	twins
gente (f.)	people
glándulas de Montgomery (f.)	Montgomery glands
glosario (m.)	glossary
gotear	leaking, to leak
goteo de leche (m.)	leaking milk
gotero (m.)	dropper
gracias	thank you
grande	big
grande	large
grano (m.)	grain
grasa (f.)	fat
gripe (f.)	flu, cold
grupo de apoyo a la lactancia (m.)	breastfeeding support group
guardar	keep, to; store, to
guardería (f.)	daycare
gustar	be pleasing, to

H

hablar	talk, to; speak, to
hacer	do, to; make, to
hasta	until
hemorragia (f.)	hemorrhage
herida (f.)	injury
hermana (f.)	sister
hermano (m.)	brother
hielo (m.)	ice
hierba (f.)	herb
hierro (m.)	iron
hija (f.)	daughter
hijo (m.)	son (child)
hinchado	engorged, swollen
hinchazón (m.)	engorgement
hipertensión (f.)	hypertension
hipertiroidismo (m.)	hyperthyroidism
hipoglicemia (f.)	hypoglycemia
hojas de col (f.)	cabbage leaves
hola	hello, hi
hombro (m.)	shoulder
hora (f.)	hour
hormona (f.)	hormone
hospital (m.)	hospital
hoy	today
huelga de lactancia (f.)	nursing strike
hundido	sunk into

I, J

implante mamario (m.)	breast implant
implantes mamarios (m.)	implants
importante	important
inclinarse hacia atrás	tilt back, to

incrementar	increase, to
infección de hongo (f.)	yeast infection
infección de hongo (f.), algodoncillo (m.)	thrush
infección del oído (f.)	ear infection
infección del pecho (f.)	breast infection
infectado	infected
inglés (m.)	English
inquieto	fussy
inquieto, molesto	upset
insertar	insert, to
insulina (f.)	insulin
intentar, tartar de	try, to
interés (m.)	interest
introducir	introduce, to
jefe (m.)	boss
jugar	play, to
juntos	together
La Liga de la Leche, Internacional (f.)	La Leche League, International
labio leporino (m.)	cleft lip
labios (m.)	lips
lactancia (f.)	breastfeeding
lactancia adoptiva (f.)	adoptive nursing
lactancia een tándem (dos bebés) (f.)	tandem nursing
lactancia exclusiva (f.)	exclusive breastfeeding
lactancia materna (f.)	breastfeeding
lactancia prolongada (f.)	extended breastfeeding
largo	long
lavaplatos (m.)	dishwasher
lavar	wash, to; clean, to
leche (f.)	milk
leche donada (f.)	donated milk
leche final (f.)	hindmilk
leche inicial (f.)	foremilk
leche materna (f.)	breastmilk
lengua (f.)	tongue
lentamente	slowly
lento, despacio	slow
letárgico	lethargic
ley (f.)	law
libra (f.)	pound
libro (m.)	book
licencia de maternidad (f.)	maternity leave
líder (m./f.)	leader
línea recta (f.)	straight line
líquido (m.)	fluid, liquid
listo	ready
llamar	call, to (by phone)
llamarse	named, to be
lleno	full
llevar	take, to; wear, to
llevar	wear, to; take, to
llorar	crying, to cry

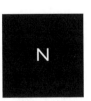

machacado	mashed
madre, mamá (f.)	mother
mamadera (f.), biberón (m.)	baby bottle
mamar	suckling
mamografía (m.)	mammogram
mancha (f.)	stain, spot
mandíbula (f.)	jaw
mano (f.)	hand
mantener	maintain, to
más que	more than
más tarde	later
masaje (m.)	massage
masaje del pecho (m.)	breast massage
masajear	massage, to
mastitis (f.)	mastitis
mayoría (f.)	majority, most
meconio (m.)	meconium
medicamento (m.), medicina (f.)	medication
mejor	better, best
mes (m.)	month
metanfetamina (f.)	crack
método de amenorea lactacional (m.)	lactational amenorrhea method
mezclar	mix, to
microondas (m.)	microwave
mililitro (m.)	milliliter (ml)
mirar	look at, to
mismo	same
mojado	wet
morder	biting, to bite
movimiento (m.)	movement
mucho	a lot
múltiples (m.)	multiples
muy	very
nacimiento (m.)	birth
nacimiento, parto (m.)	childbirth
nariz (f.)	nose
nariz contra el pezón	nose to nipple
necesario	necessary
necesidades especiales (f.)	special needs
necesitar	need, to
nieto (m.), nieta (f.)	grandchild
ningún	none, no
niño (m.)/niña (f.)	child
niño pequeño (m.)	toddler
no usar	do not use
noche (f.)	night
normal	normal
normalmente	normally, usually
número (m.)	number
número de teléfono (m.)	telephone number
nutricionista (m./f.)	nutritionist
nutritivo	nutritious

obesidad (f.)	obesity
obligar	obligate, to; force, to; require, to
oferta y demanda	supply and demand
oficina (f.)	office
ofrecer	offer, to
oído (m.)	ear (inside)
oír	hear, to
olor a jabón (m.)	soapy smell
onza (f.)	ounce
oreja (f.)	ear (outside)
orina (f.)	urine
otra vez	again
otro	other
oxitocina (f.)	oxytocin
padre, papá (m.)	father
padres (m.)	parents
pagar	pay, to
paladar hendido (m.)	cleft palate
pañal mojado (m.)	wet diaper
pañal sucio (m.)	dirty diaper
pañal, pamper (m.)	diaper
pañalitis (f.)	diaper rash
panza (f.), barriga (f.)	tummy
panza con panza	tummy-to-tummy
papel (m.)	paper
parecer	look like, to
pareja (f.)	partner, a pair
pasar, ocurrir	happen, to; occur, to
pastilla anticonceptiva (f.)	birth control pill
pecho, seno (m.)	breast, chest
pediatra (m./f.)	pediatrician
pegarse al pecho, agarrar	latch onto, to
peligroso	dangerous
pequeño	small
perder peso, rebajar	losing weight, to lose weight
pérdida de peso (f.)	weight loss
perfecto	perfect
período menstrual (m.)	menstrual period
períodos de alimentación frecuente (m.)	cluster feeding
períodos de succión rápida (m.)	sucking bursts
pero	but
pesado	heavy
pesar	weigh, to
peso (m.)	weight
peso al nacer (m.)	birth weight
pez (m.)	fish
pezón (m.)	nipple
pezonera (f.)	nipple shield
pezones adoloridos (m.)	sore nipples
pezones invertidos (m.)	inverted nipples
pezones perforados (m.)	pierced nipples
pezones planos (m.)	flat nipples

pezones retraídos, pezones hundidos (m.)	retracted nipples
picante	hot, spicy
piel (f.)	skin
piel con piel	skin-to-skin
piezas (f.)	parts
placenta (f.)	placenta
plástico	plastic
plátano (m.)	plantain
platicar	chat, to
poco	a little
poco a poco	gradually
poder	be able, to
poner	put, to; place, to
por favor	please
posición (f.)	hold
posición (f.)	position
posición de cuna (f.)	cradle hold
posición de cuna cruzada (f.)	cross-cradle hold
posición de fútbol americano/sandía/ lateral debajo del brazo (f.)	football hold
posición de lado (f.)	side lying hold
posición vertical (f.)	uphill
práctica (f.)	practice
pregunta (f.)	question
prematuro	premature
prenderse	attach, to (to the breast), latch onto
preocupado	worried
preocuparse	worry, to
prepararse	prepare oneself, to
presión (f.)	pressure
primer, primero	first
primo (m.)	cousin
principalmente	mostly, mainly
probablemente	probably
problema (m.)	problem
producir	produce, to
producir leche	make milk, to
productos lácteos (m.)	dairy
progesterona (f.)	progesterone
programación de comidas, imposición de un horario (f.)	scheduling
prolactina (f.)	prolactin
pronto	soon
propio	own
proteína (f.)	protein
provision (f.)	supply, back-up
próximo	next
puerco (m.)	pork
puré de (m.), en forma de puré	pureed
que causa gases	gassy
quedar	stay, to
querer	want, to
quitarse	come off, to; take off, to

Q

rápidamente	quickly
rápido	fast
reacción (f.)	reaction
reaccionar	react, to
rechazo del pecho (m.)	breast refusal
recibir	receive, to
recién nacido (m.)	newborn
recomendar	recommend, to
reducir	reduce, to; lower, to
reflejo de eyección de la leche (m.), bajada (f.)	letdown
refrigerador (m.)	refrigerator
regresar	return, to; go back, to
regreso (m.)	return
regulador (m.)	dial
regularmente	regularly
regurgitar, escupir	spit up, to
relactación (f.)	relactation
reloj (m.)	clock, watch
reloj (m.)	watch, clock
repetir	repeat, to
reposicionar al bebé	repositioning baby
resfriado (m.)	cold (illness)
reto (m.)	challenge
retraso del crecimiento (m.)	failure to thrive
rico	rich
rojo	red
ronchas (f.), salpullido (m.), sarpullido (m.)	rash
saber	know, to (a fact)
sacaleches (m.), bomba (f.), tiraleches (m.)	breast pump
sacarle el gas al bebé	burp your baby, to
sacarse (la leche)	express, to; pump, to
sala de recién nacidos (f.)	nursery (hospital)
salud (f.)	health
sangrar	bleeding, to bleed
sangre (f.)	blood
sano, saludable	healthy
seguir	continue, to; follow, to
segundo	second
senos grandes (m.)	large breasts
sentarse	sit, to; sit down, to
sentimiento (m.)	feeling
sentir, sentirse	feel, to (an emotion)
si	if, whether
sí	yes
siempre	always
significar	mean, to
simplemente	simply
síndrome de Down (m.)	Down Syndrome

síndrome de muerte infantil súbita (SMIS) (m.)	SIDS (Sudden Infant Death Syndrome)
síndrome de ovario policístico (m.)	polycystic ovary syndrome (PCOS)
síndrome de Sheehan (m.)	Sheehan's Syndrome
síntoma (m.)	symptom
sistema (m.)	system
sistema de lactancia suplementaria (m.)	supplemental nursing system
sobreproducción de leche (f.)	oversupply
sobrina (f.)	niece
sobrino (m.)	nephew
sólo	only, just
solución (f.)	solution
sonido (m.)	sound
sonidos de chasquidos (m.)	clicking sounds
sostén con varillas, sostén con aros (m.)	underwire
sostener	hold, to
soya (f.)	soy
suavemente	gently
subida de la leche (f.)	coming in (milk)
succión (f.)	suction
succionar	suck, to; suction, to
sucio	dirty
suegra (f.)	mother-in-law
suficiente	enough
suficiente	sufficient
sugerencia (f.)	suggestion
sugerir	suggest, to
suplementar	supplement, to
suplementos (m.)	supplements
taburete (m.)	stool (furniture)
tamaño	size
también	also
tan	so (so long)
tanto	so much
tapón (m.)	plug
taza (f.), vaso (m.)	cup
tazón (m.)	bowl
técnica (f.)	technique
teléfono (m.)	telephone
temperatura ambiente (f.)	room temperature
tener	have, to
tener hambre	hungry, to be
tener sed	thirsty, to be
terminar	finish, to
tía (f.)	aunt
tibia	warm
tiempo	time (chronological)
tierno	tender
tío (m.)	uncle
tocar	touch, to
todavía	still, yet

T

U, V, W

toma (f.), comida de pecho (f.), lactada (f.)	feeding
tomar	drink, to
tomar	take, to; drink, to
tomas nocturnas (f.)	night feedings
trabajo (m.)	work
tragar	gulping, to gulp
tragar	swallow, to
tratamiento quiropráctico (m.)	chiropractic treatment
trigo (m.)	wheat
trillizos (m.)	triplets
tubería (f.)	tubing (for pump)
unidad de cuidados intensivos neonatal (f.)	NICU (Neonatal Intensive Care Unit)
usar	use, to
utilizar	utilize, to
vacuna (f.)	vaccination, vaccine
vasospasmo (m.)	vasospasm
vegetal (m.)	vegetable
velocidad (f.)	speed
verdad (f.)	true
verde	green
vez, veces (f.)	time, times (occurrences)
virus VIH (m.)	HIV virus
Vitamina D (f.)	Vitamin D
vomitar	throwing up
vomitar	vomiting, to vomit
WIC	WIC

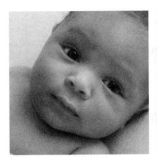

INDEX

ABOUT THE AUTHORS

DIANA B. GLICK

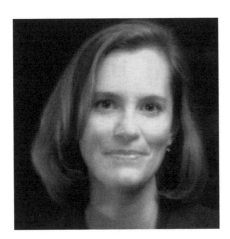

Diana B. Glick received her Bachelor's Degree from Mount Holyoke College and holds a Master's Degree in Spanish and a *Juris Doctor* from the University of California, Davis. In addition, she holds a certificate in Medical Interpreting from the University of Massachusetts, Amherst. Ms. Glick taught Spanish for Medical Professionals and volunteered as a medical interpreter with a family practice clinic. She currently practices law and lives with her husband and daughter in California.

TANYA M. LIEBERMAN

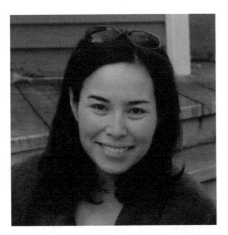

Tanya M. Lieberman, IBCLC, is a lactation consultant who works in hospital and pediatric office settings. She completed the University of California, San Diego, lactation consultant course and the University of California, Los Angeles, lactation educator course. She also writes and records podcasts for a popular breastfeeding website, the Motherwear Breastfeeding Blog. Prior to becoming a lactation consultant, she was senior education and fiscal policy staff for the California Legislature and Governor. She lives with her husband and two children in Massachusetts.

ORDERING INFORMATION

HALE PUBLISHING, L.P.

■ ■ ■

1712 N. FOREST ST.
AMARILLO, TEXAS 79106
USA

■ ■ ■

8:00 AM TO 5:00 PM CST

■ ■ ■

ONLINE ORDERS
WWW.IBREASTFEEDING.COM

OTHER
HALE PUBLISHING
TITLES

MEDICATIONS AND MOTHERS' MILK

◼◼◼

MINI MEDICATIONS AND MOTHERS' MILK

◼◼◼

NONPRESCRIPTION DRUGS FOR THE
BREASTFEEDING MOTHER

◼◼◼

HALE & HARTMANN'S TEXTBOOK OF
HUMAN LACTATION